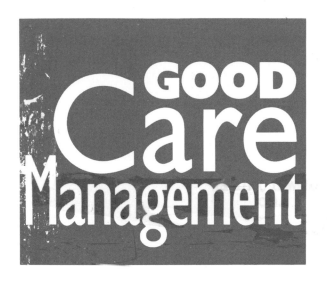

A GUIDE TO SETTING UP
AND MANAGING
A RESIDENTIAL HOME

Jenyth Worsley

*In loving memory of Victoria Talbot Rice
(1897–1990) who taught me so much about
the wisdom of age*

**CORNWALL COLLEGE
LRC**

© 1992 Jenyth Worsley
Published by ACE Books
Age Concern England
1268 London Road
London SW16 4ER

Editor Lee Bennett
Design Eugenie Dodd
Copy Preparation Vinnette Marshall
Production Marion Peat
Typeset by Grosvenor Press, Portsmouth
Printed and bound by Ebenezer Baylis, Worcester

A catalogue record for this book is
available from the British Library.

ISBN 0-86242-104-7

As stated in the Introduction, some of the information in this book relates to legislation not yet fully in
force. Although great care has been taken in the
compilation of the book, Age Concern England and
the author cannot accept responsibility for any errors
or omissions.

Contents

Sponsor's Foreword

Esso is delighted to be able to mark the Golden Jubilee of Age Concern through sponsorship of *Good Care Management*.

Esso has a strong commitment to the provision of high quality and cost efficient services. We recognise the importance of good management practice in delivering these services to our customers. We are particularly pleased therefore to sponsor *Good Care Management* which aims to enable the proprietors and managers of residential homes to improve their commercial management, to be in full compliance with relevant legislation and to pursue the highest standards of good management practice.

Sir Archibald Forster
Chairman and Chief Executive
Esso UK plc

About the Author

Good Care Management is the second skills training resource book which Jenyth Worsley has written for Age Concern England. She is also the author of *Taking Good Care: A Handbook for Care Assistants*. Other subjects she has written about include the performing arts, negotiation and working in nursing and teaching for the Careers and Occupational Information Centre, Department of Employment. She has also contributed articles to the *Oxford Children's Encyclopedia*, published by the Oxford University Press.

She earlier worked in BBC radio as a producer and writer for a wide range of programmes including a ten-part series on business studies, 'Listen with Mother', 'Story Time', and drama features for Radio 3 and 4. She has directed for fringe theatre and is currently writing a novel on colonial Africa.

Jenyth is active in the Society of Authors and sings with a chamber choir in Oxford.

Acknowledgments

I should like to express my gratitude and appreciation to the following people and organisations for their help in the preparation of this book:

Angela Avis, Professional Head of District Nursing, Oxfordshire; Symon Clarke, Social Services Department, Kingston-upon-Thames; Verena Mitchell, Principal Inspector and Peter Perman Howe, Team Manager, Oxfordshire Social Services Department; Carmel Creighton, Evenlode House; Bill Bowley, Newland House; Janet Walsh, St Anne's Residential Home; Tim Geddy, St Luke's Residential Home, together with their residents and staff.

For their advice and comments: C Paul Brearley, Director, Disabled Living Foundation; Des Kelly, Deputy General Secretary, Social Care Association; Professor Grimley Evans, Department of Geriatric Medicine, Oxford University; Dr Rebecca Mather; Dr Anne Roberts; Sheila Scott, Secretary, National Care Homes Association; Gordon McLaurin, Anchor Housing Association; Veronica Jones, Age Concern Training; Evelyn McEwen, Divisional Director (Services), Age Concern England.

I much appreciate being able to draw on research by: Anchor Housing Association; the Wakefield Social Services Department; Dr G Cherry, Department of Dermatology, The Slade Hospital, Oxford, for guidelines on the treatment of chronic ulcers. Thanks also to Gemma Jones for the programme on dementia management, as outlined in Appendix 2.

Finally, my thanks to Linda Coverdale for her assistance in research and in proof-reading the manuscript.

Jenyth Worsley
January 1992

Introduction

There are more people than ever living into old age. Many lead an active life well into their eighties, some are cared for at home by relatives and friends, while others have some support from the community or voluntary organisations. In Great Britain about 3 per cent (263,000) of those over 65 live in residential care homes, and about half of these (131,200) are over 85.

Choosing to run a Home for older people as your own business or managing one for someone else involve the same challenges. You will probably have worked with older people before and found how very different they are, one from another, while life has given them so many different experiences. You will want to make their care your first priority, to make them comfortable in your Home, to respect their rights as individuals and ensure that your staff are alert to the needs of each particular resident.

Many of the legal, administrative and business problems faced by new owners are also common to managers of private, local authority and voluntary homes. The same skills are needed in how to choose and train your staff, how to delegate and allocate the work, how you run a household for twenty four hours a day, interlinking night and day staff and domestic staff – and how you interact with the community medical, nursing and social services.

This book will discuss all these areas and is designed to offer guidance to managers and owners of private, voluntary and local authority homes. It draws on the research, experience and good practice of people and organisations involved in making good care work and in developing management and business skills. It also tells you about the changes taking place as a result of recent legislation which you will need to consider before setting up a Home and how these will affect the way Homes will be managed.

THINK IT THROUGH CAREFULLY

You should not underestimate the problems you will have to face in setting up and running a residential home. It takes time, abundant energy, all the skills you can call on in caring for individual residents, discussing issues with their relatives and supporting your staff. You will need to manage your resources prudently, ensure that your administration is efficient and that your own and your staff's training needs are kept to the forefront in planning the timetable.

Good business practice

On the business side, planning and good financial management are vital to keep the Home running, to provide a living for the owner and to assess current and future needs. Good book-keeping and an experienced accountant are essential. There are a number of organisations which give practical help and advice to businesses. They include Training and Enterprise Councils, local authority business development units and local Chambers of Commerce.

Help from the inspectorate

Local authority independent inspection units are a major source of advice and help for managers. The units are responsible for registration and inspection of nearly all residential care homes. The inspection team has wide experience of different kinds of Home and is particularly concerned with the quality of care.

Back-up from the community

At first, running a Home successfully may seem a daunting task. You are not only running a business, but that business is concerned with some of the most vulnerable people in our society. So it is important to remember that the Home owner or manager is not alone in caring for the residents. They are also the concern of the inspection team and many other people involved in providing support such as the primary health care team.

In addition you will find local community support from religious and voluntary groups and from the friends and family of residents. Many Homes also have an advisory committee drawn from interested people in the community, who can give advice on all kinds of issues from refurbishing rooms to whether to diversify by offering short-term respite care.

Training for everyone

This is the key to the successful running of any organisation. It should include initial induction for new staff members and on-going skills training and personal development for management and staff. Many training organisations and local colleges run sandwich, part-time and full-time courses leading to vocational and National Vocational Qualifications. Some of these agencies and Age Concern England offer short courses in a variety of different areas – for example, on dementia, managing continence, and the characteristics of ageing. Local authorities will, increasingly, offer courses for a fee.

KEY POINTS

- Running a good residential home requires a combination of good business management, care skills and staff/personnel management.
- Good advice and support will help you take advantage of new opportunities.
- The best care comes when management and staff are well trained and confident in their work.
- You should aim to provide the best quality of life possible for each resident in your Home.

DEVELOPMENTS IN COMMUNITY CARE

The last few years have seen considerable research into what type of care should be provided for people of all ages with care needs. Many of the proposals were incorporated in the Government White Paper, *Caring for People*, and the National Health Service and Community Care Act, 1990. The changes are being implemented in stages, and it is unlikely that all the details of administration and funding will be known until the new system is up and running. It will therefore be very important for Home managers to keep in touch with these changes; and even more important for those considering setting up a Home to work out how far the changes will make their plans viable. The proposed date for full implementation (at the time of going to print) is April 1993.

Population changes

One of the predisposing factors behind the changes in community care is the growing number of older people in the population who will require residential care or support from the community in order to remain in their own homes.

It is estimated that by the year 2,000 in Great Britain there will be almost 4.5 million people over the age of 75 and almost 1.1 million over 85. A further relevant factor is that more and more women in their forties and fifties are now returning to the workforce. This may mean a drop in informal carers available to look after their relatives or friends.

There are also the implications of certain diseases such as Alzheimer's and Parkinson's Disease. People who suffer from these and other conditions will need a great deal of expensive care whether they live in residential homes or in their own homes in the community.

Community care plans

The White Paper and the Act are designed to promote and improve the quality of all care provision. Local authorities are required to produce annual community care plans which must show the result of their assessment of the needs of people living in their area and explain what services will be on offer to meet those needs. The plans must be produced in consultation with users of services and their carers and with organisations representing them. There must also be consultation with other statutory agencies and bodies providing health, housing and other services. Clearly, you, as a residential care manager or owner, have an opportunity here to contribute to local planning.

The plans will cover targets, arrangements for assessment, how assessment will be made, how quality care is to be monitored and ways of increasing choice in the kind of care being offered. The plans will also show how the authority proposes to stimulate the private and voluntary sector in the provision of all forms of care – in people's own homes and in residential and nursing homes. The plans will be examined each year by the Social Services Inspectorate which is part of the Department of Health.

In some areas, where there is currently little independent provision, local authorities will be expected to encourage the development of services other than those they already provide. There will be real opportunities for the independent sector to expand existing or develop new services. These plans will hold the key to the future. Home owners will need to watch the policy developments and strategies of their own authority carefully and enter into discussions about where they could increase their contribution to care services.

Inspection

As mentioned earlier, local authority inspectors are a source of help to managers. They are responsible for registering, inspecting and monitoring residential care and advising management how to provide all-round quality. The inspectors are now in 'arms length' inspection units within the social services department, which must be independent from the delivery of services directly provided by the authority including the management of Homes.

At the moment Homes with Royal Charters and very small Homes do not have to be registered and inspected. However, it is proposed sometime in 1992 to introduce simplified registration procedures for Homes catering for three or fewer residents. If necessary the inspection team would also be able to check on such Homes. They are also now inspecting the local authority's own Homes, which will mean that some will need improvements to bring their standard up to that which is required of private and voluntary homes.

Funding care

There will also be changes in how care is funded. From April 1993 there will be a shift from grants paid to individual men and women through Income Support to funds transferred by the Government to local authorities and administered through their social services departments. The sum will vary from authority to authority and will be included with the general funds provided by the Government through the revenue support grant. Age Concern England produces Factsheets on funding residential care which will keep you up to date from year to year as the situation changes (see p 178).

Residents who are in Homes before 1993 and who need Income Support will continue to be funded in this way, and those whose capital drops below the limit of eligibility (currently £8,000) will also have access to this assistance if their income falls below the level at which Income Support can be paid.

Assessment

Until April 1993 anyone who wishes to go into a Home can claim Income Support without an assessment of their need. After April 1993, all that will change. Anyone needing financial help to pay for their care will need to apply to the local social services department for an assessment. Each local authority will set up its own criteria for eligibility, so it is not easy to generalise about who will be eligible for assessment for any particular form of care. In the assessment procedure, a range of options will be discussed. Going into a Home may only be one of them. As older people generally want to stay in their own homes, every effort will be made to bring services to them first. As this is also generally regarded as the best use of limited resources, it is possible that only very frail people will be assessed as needing full-time residential care.

If finally it is decided that a residential home is the best option, social workers are likely to be the key professionals involved in admitting someone to your Home. You will work closely with them while the resident is settling into the Home.

People will not have to be assessed if they don't wish to be, and if they can arrange their own care. However, attention will need to be paid to the form of assessment which will be used for residents who enter Homes in this way after 1993 and who might subsequently need additional financial help to pay for their place in the Home.

Packages of care

Under the White Paper, local authorities should be aiming for a 'mixed economy of care' to meet the needs of their local communities, as identified in their community care plans. Those who assess the need for care and who purchase services should ideally have their activities separated from those who provide services within the social services department. It is the

Government's intention that there should be fair competition between those providing residential care – whether it is in a local authority, a private or a voluntary home.

Local authorities are likely to be running fewer residential homes of their own, either closing them completely or selling or transferring them to an external management group. They will therefore be purchasing care from independent providers either on a case-by-case basis or through block contracts with a variety of providers. Authorities may ask Home managers or owners to tender for contracts, and Homes which can show a quality product at a competitive price will have the edge over the others. Owners will need to look into the implications of the different types of contract very carefully and are urged to get advice from a professional association (see p 164).

Terms of contract

Every contract between local authorities and Home proprietors or managers will set out in detail the obligations of both sides. Some block contracts may specify exactly how many places the authority wishes to reserve, but others may only ask for a call on places. The terms may also vary: owners may be obliged to accept any resident the authority wishes to place in the Home, or they may have the right to be consulted and the right to refuse admission. Contracts should also specify the circumstances when the Home owner will need to raise prices – for example, when dependency levels of residents change. It is important to check these points when you are negotiating contracts, and to make sure that they can be altered if the terms do not prove to be workable in practice.

If you accept residents referred by the social services department, you will be expected to conform to the series of quality standards set down in the contract which will specify how these will be monitored and met in the care package. Where authorities give contracts for individual places, you will also have to negotiate with the prospective resident or his or her advocate and the social services before a contract is drawn up.

Once the resident has agreed to come and live in your Home, you will not only be expected to support them in managing their daily lives but you may also have to work with relatives, friends and others who are involved in their lives.

16

KEY POINTS

- Local authorities must draw up community care plans in consultation with users and providers of care services.

- The independent sector is being encouraged to provide more and different forms of care.

- Homes, including those run by the local authority, will be inspected by a unit which is independent from the authority's own provision.

- After 1993 local authorities will be responsible for funding any new resident who needs financial support from the State, and this will only be forthcoming after an assessment of need.

- Some Homes will be offered contracts by authorities sometimes through a block booking of beds. Other Homes may choose to remain independent of these arrangements.

- Local authority homes may need to improve the quality of care they provide to bring it up to the standard required for private and voluntary homes.

Starting Out

During the past few years more and more people have opted to start their own businesses. Many have succeeded, although few of them may have realised what they were taking on, and many would probably have backed away if they could have gazed into a crystal ball!

Most people, when deciding to go into business for themselves, have a skill they feel could probably be better utilised by working for themselves, rather than being adapted to suit an employer. It does not necessarily follow, however, that an experienced nurse will be able to start up a successful business running a residential home – or that a successful hotel-keeper can provide good quality care. Whatever your background, before starting out in any venture, it is always wise to take time over planning, and to take advantage of as much advice as possible.

Other factors you will need to consider in preparing yourself to own or run a Home are:

- a business plan
- your marketing strategy
- choosing the right property
- how to register a Home
- legal requirements

In this chapter we cover these areas of concern for someone deciding to set up and run a residential home.

PERSONAL PROFILE

Setting up and running a residential home should not be entered into lightly. There are other ways of making a quicker return on your investment. Many people who decide to make Home management their way of life have had professional contact with older people in the course of their career – nurses, doctors, social workers are among them.

Owner 'When I was a nurse, I always preferred to be on the medical wards because there were more elderly people there. I always think it was because of my grandmother. I've great memories of her as a child and she was a wonderful person. She taught me so much.'

But Home owners come in other guises. A successful chef who at one time ran his own restaurant now looks after a private home in the West Country. A former business woman from Edinburgh has found satisfaction in the care she now gives to the 120 people in her Home.

Partner 'I thought I would be always totally involved in the finance and didn't want to be involved in the care side, but it's incredible what I'm getting out of it. I know all the staff - it's like a vibrant family that is constantly changing and I'm getting far more from it than I've actually put in – though I have to admit that for the last two years I have worked a seven day week, and normally I am not home before seven or eight in the evening.'

When deciding to take the plunge and 'go it alone', whatever line you choose, many aspects ought to be considered. Do you have the support of your family? Do you have a clear idea of where you intend the venture to take you? Are you the right sort of person to run your own business? Do you have the necessary qualifications and experience, including a minimum of one year managing a Home at senior level?

Your goals

This is the stage to consider your goals in life, your reasons for wanting to run a home, and the personal qualities and management skills which you will need. Ask yourself the following questions.

– What do I want to get out of life?

- What would be my principles in running a Home?
- Am I self-disciplined?
- Am I ready to put in the necessary hours?
- Can I cope under stress?
- Will I give in if the going gets tough?
- Can I learn from my mistakes without getting disheartened?
- Am I aware of the risks to myself and others?
- Do I have proper back-up?
- Have I the necessary management and leadership skills?
- How do I feel about others doing the work their way, and not my way?
- Do I know the market?
- Am I able to provide a quality service?
- Can I make a commitment for at least five years?

If your answers to these questions are positive, some of the problems that will inevitably crop up will not come as a surprise.

IMPROVE YOUR MANAGEMENT SKILLS

It is a sad and avoidable fact that many businesses fail because there is no overall financial plan and strict accounts are not kept. Running a Home means that there always has to be a balance between business and Home, and managers need to keep a strict check on all the different budgets – household, health care, maintenance, food and wages.

A leading bank has drawn up some useful advice for new proprietors, as listed below:

- Make time to attend courses, seminars and functions where you meet other people in your field.
- Regularly read the literature of your professional association as well as the weekly and monthly care press.
- Listen to and watch 'small business' programmes on radio and TV.
- Talk to and seek advice from professionals.

A business plan

Thorough planning in financial control, client profile and staffing levels is the first priority and should be done before you even pick up the phone to talk to an estate agent. Once you have formulated some ideas, you need to set them out clearly in a business plan.

Basically, a business plan is the first stage in forward planning. It will show clearly the aims of the Home, how it is likely to grow and how you will market it. A business plan gives a good opportunity to examine your own ideas, ideals, hopes and fears. It provides evidence that you have given careful thought to the undertaking and will certainly be required by banks, or anyone who is considering giving you financial backing to fund the purchase of premises, convert the property, etc.

At this stage you will only be able to make a very provisional business plan, but, nevertheless, it is an essential document. After completing your plan, see what questions you then need to ask and arrange to talk to a variety of sources of help.

Getting help from others

Banks – small business section

Most banks run these with a dedicated small business manager. He or she will give advice on any aspect of running a business, and will provide leaflets and back-up material free of charge. Their advice will be general, but is nonetheless valuable as a background canvas to give you a framework to fill in with more detail as your ideas develop.

Sole Proprietor 'Whilst the small business manager I approached regarding my new venture listened politely and offered some encouragement, I did feel rather at first that he couldn't offer specific advice. On thinking about it later, I realised that in many ways I had more idea of what was required in my field than he did – but at least I went home with a handful of literature, which in the event proved very useful.

'I hadn't actually given any thought to a business plan but the booklets went into a lot of detail. I started to feel more able to write a plan and what was expected out of it. I became a lot more confident as my ideas began to take on a more solid shape.'

Advice from other organisations

There are a number of agencies which provide excellent advice for people who are setting up or running a small business. They include:

Department of Trade and Industry Small Firms Service - for London only.

The Rural Development Commission (RDC).

Training and Enterprise Councils (TECs).

Local authority business development units.

Local Chambers of Commerce.

Professional associations.

Details and addresses of these organisations or agencies are given in 'Further Information' (see p 164).

Raising finance

Business start-up means taking risks, and usually the first is backing your ideas with capital of your own.

Partner 'To raise the finance, I put together a business plan and remortgaged my house to match the offer of £30,000 from an organisation willing to provide a "soft" loan for projects of this type. This was seven years ago, so it was quite a lot at the time. It meant everything was risked - absolutely everything, to such a point that I used to come home at night and, as the costs of conversion of the property ran higher and higher, my little girl would say, "Have you had a good day, Mummy, and have we still got the house?".'

This manager is referring to a time when interest rates were low. When they increase, the risk of losing everything in a long-term venture is even higher, and has to be assessed extremely carefully.

Your marketing strategy

Marketing is very important in the success or failure of any venture, new or old. Marketing has two parts: finding out about your potential clients and deciding what is the best way to attract them to your Home.

Partner 'Before we even raised the money, we had to carry out our own market research, which took us two years whilst I was doing other work. We phoned every authority in every areas, we phoned existing residential and nursing home owners, and gradually put together a picture of how the numbers had risen and the need had increased over the last ten years, and how they saw the trends for the next ten years.'

Those are some of the points to be considered in your own research, and again, it is worth spending some time considering your marketing strategy before you embark on time-consuming research.

– Do you understand the market you are in? Define it in a written statement.

– Where do you see the majority of your residents coming from in terms of social class, ethnic group, income, type of disability and so on?

– Are you aiming mostly for the privately funded or the publicly funded resident? What are the financial and care implications for your choice?

– Have you thought about having residents with specific conditions or from certain ethnic groups?

– What are the demographic changes in the population for your area now and for the future?

– How many Homes are there in your area, and what is the demand for places?

– Have you established good contacts with the social and health services?

– Is your service right for your perceived customer group?

– Will it be up to social services inspectorate current and future requirements? Is it what you think they want or what you know they want?

– How do you propose to make yourself known and to sell your services to clients?

– Will you attract staff in areas of perceived need?

– Have you talked to people who might recommend your Home or refer residents to investigate the service you propose to offer?

– Do you know what is happening in relation to competition, economic factors and what financial subsidies are likely to be available for people in your market?

– Have you looked at ways in which your business might develop in future, as mentioned in the chapter 'Branching Out'?

The answers to some of these questions will be suggested in this book, but only you can find out about the competition – how much other Homes are charging and what they are offering. Do not be put off by the number of people offering similar services to the ones you intend to provide – be confident that you give better value for money and have something unique to offer.

Choice of property

While you are doing your research, look at properties and compare prices in different areas. Having decided on the right location, the next step is to search for a suitable property. Take time to select with care, bearing in mind the aims of your business plan. It may be more economical in the long run to buy a site which seems dauntingly large rather than to take on an established business. Ask yourself the following questions:

–   What type of property will best suit the needs of the residents I plan to give a home to, and can I afford it?
–   Will there be staff available in the vicinity, especially for night work?
–   What about off-peak transport to and from the Home for staff members?
–   How much conversion will the property require before registration and to fulfil fire and health and safety regulations?
–   What are the costs of conversion and are they within my capital budget?

REGISTERING THE HOME

At this planning stage, you will also need to find out as much as you can about all the legal aspects of setting up a residential home and to make sure you are able to satisfy all the statutory requirements. In some areas these are co-ordinated by the registration officer of the independent inspection unit. In others, you will have to liaise separately with individual local authority departments.

The Registered Homes Act, 1984 (amended, 1991), requires residential homes in the private or voluntary sectors (apart from those with Crown Immunity) which provide personal care and board for four people and above to be registered by the local authority. As explained in the

'Introduction', this will be operated by the 'arms length' inspection units set up in each authority under the NHS and Community Care Act, 1990. They will issue guidelines for procedures in their own areas, subject to the requirements of the Act.

It is proposed sometime in 1992 to introduce simplified registration procedures for 'small Homes', those catering for three or fewer residents. If necessary, the inspection unit would also be able to check on such Homes.

One of the main purposes behind the registration system is to monitor standards of care in residential homes and to raise those that fall short. The Act requires the 'person in control' – this person usually being the owner – to apply for registration. Where there is a separate manager, both people should be registered.

Principal inspection officer 'If you are thinking of setting up a Home you need to know what registration is about. The first thing I suggest to prospective owners is that they obtain the pack which local authorities have prepared for new Home owners. It includes guidance notes on the Registered Homes Act, the regulations, a copy of the Code of Practice, *Home Life*, a book on administration of drugs, staffing, and guidance on all the other local authority regulations including fire regulations, health and safety, etc. Finally the pack includes an application form and a list of all the other Homes in the area that are registered. New owners need to know all the responsibilities placed on them as a registered person, including the training of their own staff.'

Registration usually covers three stages.
1   An inspection of plans and premises, after which the proprietor is told exactly what further work must be done and approved before registration is granted.
2   While this further work is carried out, the owner and the inspectorate discuss matters of client profile, staffing, etc.
3   Finally, discussions take place on how the owner is actually going to run the Home.

While researching how to set up a Home, you may discover that some Homes are registered to provide both residential and nursing care and are dually registered. The nursing home element has to be registered by the district health authority for the higher levels of nursing care involved. If you are intending to provide this, discuss your plans with the district health authority.

The application

The actual application form provides evidence that you have thought carefully and seriously about all aspects of setting up a Home. The book *Home Life* (details on page 168) gives very helpful guidance in a number of areas, including the following:

- A statement of the aims and objectives of the Home, including the philosophy of care and the type and standard of support available.
- Personal details, including qualifications and experience, references and fitness (if appropriate) of the owner, manager and all staff. (A Home run by a company will also have to submit these details.)
- A declaration of the owner's/manager's other business interests.
- Details of the Home, including its address, the accommodation available for staff and residents and the proposed date of opening.
- Copies of the plans of the building, details of equipment and facilities.
- The number, sex and category of residents.
- Draft brochures, showing services to be provided.
- Draft contracts for residents and staff.
- Draft job descriptions.
  Charges to residents.
- Other details (arrangements for medical and dental treatment, the handling of medicines, staff rotas).

Any person who is setting up a Home is obliged to disclose a criminal record. Some offences have a 'rehabilitation period' after which the sentence is considered to be 'spent', ie wiped off the record. However, certain sentences because of their severity can never become spent. These include life imprisonment, sentences for more than 30 months and detention during 'Her Majesty's Pleasure'. Exceptions are also made for members of certain professions whatever the sentence, and these include occupations concerned with the running of an establishment which is required to be registered under the Registered Homes Act, 1984.

The inspector will need to satisfy himself that the care to be offered in a Home is along the lines outlined above and also in the Department of Health practice guidelines. Ways in which managers and owners can demonstrate good practice are outlined in more detail throughout this book.

Applications should be accompanied by the appropriate fee. If registration is granted, owners pay an annual fee, due one month after registration. If it is refused, the principal inspector has to inform the owner in writing. The owner or manager can then appeal to the local authority in the first place, and then to a registered homes tribunal. The most common reasons for refusal of registration or deregistration of a Home after inspection are:

- The unfitness of the proprietor, in the opinion of the inspector, to run a Home.
- Inadequate staffing levels, and inaccurate or incomplete record keeping.
- Unsuitable premises.
- Evidence of racial discrimination or of uncaring staff attitudes leading to neglect of residents.

Inspection

After registration is granted to a Home, the authority has the power to make inspections at any time – with a minimum of twice a year. Inspection is intended to be positive, and to create a working partnership between the Home and the inspectorate. If an inspector believes that changes are necessary, he or she will negotiate with the Home owner. You will find further details on inspection on pages 139–142.

Other legal requirements

Planning and building regulations

When you have found a property which seems to fit the bill, there are several things to consider. If the property was originally an ordinary family house, and you wish to use it as a residential home for more than six people, you will need planning permission to alter its status. This is done through your local planning authority and may take some time. Planning committees meet about every six weeks depending on the routine in individual areas.

When applying for planning permission for a change of use to your property, be sure to ask about future development plans for the area that interests you. These could have a dramatic effect on your business, one way or another.

It is also important at this stage to have the property valued and surveyed by an independent chartered surveyor as well as to take advice from an architect who is experienced in similar conversions. This will ensure that the price you have been asked to pay is fair, and that you are aware of any potential problems regarding the structure of the building before you sign on the dotted line.

Owner 'It's an elegant old house, built around 1866. There are lovely walks even within the building, you could really walk until you tire yourself out with the nice long corridors. One of our residents, Nessie, takes a walk every day – she does ten up and down from the front door down to the back and that's her exercise. The rooms are a nice size and the ceilings are very high, which of course gives it air. There are lovely grounds now to walk all around the building and no steps to cope with, it's all slopes – good for wheelchairs as well.'

Health and safety

Today more and more emphasis is being placed on health and safety, and inevitably the number of rules and regulations are growing. Before opening your Home, you will have to satisfy the environmental health department of your local authority that you will be running a safe, well planned establishment.

Environmental health officers will come and inspect your Home and ask for various certificates to be provided, depending on the equipment, etc you own. They will check on all aspects of basic safety in the Home, as well as special requirements for elderly residents. Where required, they report their findings to the registration officer and to the manager.

In the planning stages you have to give a great deal of thought to the provision of wide doorways, wheelchair ramps, bath rails, non-slip floors in toilets and bathrooms, lifts, air-conditioning, etc. The first points mentioned are straight-forward good practice. Once you venture into the area of lifts and air conditioning, the environmental health officer will need to see evidence of regular testing – every six months in the case of lifts.

Having a policy

If you have more than five employees, you will need to draw up a health and safety policy in line with the Health and Safety at Work Act, 1974. This basically ensures that all employees know what is expected of them regarding health and safety matters, and can save time and argument in the event of a disagreement. Your employees should be fully trained in carrying out the policy, and copies of the Health and Safety Executive approved poster and leaflets should be kept somewhere easily accessible to everyone. These are available from HMSO. All staff should know exactly what to do in the event of an accident.

NOTE   Managers of Homes with fewer than five employees should check with the local Health and Safety Executive, as these Homes may in the future need to display a policy.

COSHH regulations

Regulations about the Control of Substances Hazardous to Health require you to list and store each and every substance you may have on the premises which could cause potential harm to residents and staff. This includes ordinary household cleaning items such as bleach and disinfectants, all the medication you keep in the Home and stronger substances, like paint stripper and weed killers.

Proprietor's responsibility

In the three areas mentioned below, proprietors have the sole responsibility for training their staff to comply with the various regulations. It is essential that a new manager is thoroughly familiar with them and ensures that staff not only know what is required but are able to carry it out in a practical way.

Food hygiene regulations

The environmental health department will also assess your methods of food handling, and will carry out regular checks. There are new regulations for food hygiene, following the 1990 Food Safety Act, which are much more stringent than previous regulations. A certificate showing that staff have qualifications in basic food hygiene issued by the Institute of Environment Health Officers should be displayed in places where food is served.

Be aware that further tests may be carried out regarding purity of the water supply in the Home and for signs of legionella, salmonella, etc. Anyone who handles food will need to be medically examined to ensure they are not carriers of these infections which could be passed on to the residents through food. You should ensure that staff are properly trained in the correct methods of food handling.

Electricity regulations

Your premises must comply with the new electricity regulations, and all electrical equipment will need to be covered by a certificate giving details of regular testing. You should make a note to have examinations carried out at six month intervals, and ensure that all records are kept up to date and available for examination by the local authority.

Fire regulations

You will also be required to comply with the fire regulations, which cover such items as smoke detectors, adequate means of escape in case of fire – more old people die from suffocation due to smoke than anything else during a fire – emergency lighting and the provision of the correct fire extinguishers.

Help from independent advisors

All the above may sound rather daunting, but your environmental health department will help and advise you where necessary. There are now also many firms that carry out health and safety audits on a regular basis, drawing your attention to any contravention of the relevant acts and regulations.

Names of companies which carry out this type of work can be found in the *Yellow Pages* listed under Safety Consultants. You should always ask them for references and take them up, to make sure that their firm is reputable. The consultants will also point out to you any dangerous practices they notice during their audits, drawing your attention to small details like fraying lino or carpets, which could become a tripping hazard for residents, worn electrical leads and larger issues such as inadequate lighting on stairs, unsanitary food handling, etc. Major problems such as COSHH assessments can also be handled by consultancy firms.

If you choose to have audits carried out on a regular basis, say twice a year, the firm of consultants you employ will be retained to answer any problems that arise between their regular visits at no extra cost. You can consult them on technical questions or ask their professional opinion on interpretation of the acts and regulations. They will also make sure that all your routine checks have been carried out to the standard required by the local authority. Their service may seem expensive at first, but you should consider whether it is cost effective.

Adequate insurance cover

You need to make sure that your insurance covers you for employer's liability. This provides cover if an employee makes a claim against a Home, for instance, if they hurt themselves moving equipment, or a pan of scalding water splashes on someone working in the kitchen. Other types of insurance which are advisable include fire, theft, loss of profits, loss of money, loss of registration and professional indemnity. It is advisable to get several quotes from insurance brokers who are members of their profession's self-regulatory organisations (the Insurance Brokers Registration Council or LAUTRO).

You should also check that residents' personal possessions are covered by insurance and that they are aware of contents policies specially designed for older people including those available from Age Concern Insurance Services (address on page 166).

You will need to maintain a record of all accidents that happen in the Home, both major and minor, whether to staff or residents. Specially designed books are available for this purpose from local authorities. It is important to fill in all the details because they may be required in medical treatment or in regard to any legal claims.

KEY POINTS

- Make a business plan.
- Take advice from as many sources as you can.
- Proper market research is crucial to the success of a new venture.
- Market research may take as long as two years.
- Always compare what you can offer with what is currently provided.

- Before registration, owners will have to satisfy the registration officer that their plans and working methods comply with Department of Health practice guidance and the code of practice *Home Life*.

- Inspections will take place at least twice a year. They are intended to promote good care in partnership with owners rather than to impose suggestions on them.

- You need to be familiar with the regulations concerning planning consent, building control and the Food Safety Act, 1990.

- Health and safety procedures are strict, and you must comply with them.

- There are specialist firms which will check out all areas covered by the Health and Safety at Work Act, 1974.

Setting up a Home

While you are looking for a suitable property for a home or while it is being converted, there are many other factors to be considered. The most import-ant is to keep in mind at all times that what you are creating is not a hotel or a hostel, but a home for men and women at the end of their lives. Good facilities, easy access to living space, well-thought-out menus, caring and knowledgeable staff are part of this. What you provide for residents will be based on your own attitudes and philosophy. The best facilities money can buy can never be a substitute for providing an atmosphere where people can live out their lives with dignity – with perhaps rather less expense but with infinitely more care.

This is the stage to decide just who will be the clientele in your Home, how you should plan the interior of the Home, the range and quality of services that residents will require and how you should recruit staff to meet their needs. In this chapter we cover these topics.

District nurse 'When new people come to a Home they leave behind so much – their house, their garden, their neighbours, their own belongings. Sometimes when I go into a Home all the furniture is regimented – every room exactly the same. And when I go in, the identity of that resident is reduced to what's on the bedside table. That seems very sad. You see the difference in places where people can take pieces of their own furniture with them. You have a sense of identity when you go in the room and the sense of a real person. When they have to share a room and they have regimented furniture although the physical care may be very good, I'm not sure about the psychological care.'

RESIDENTS' NEEDS

You have already decided to offer residential care for older people, but there are many target groups. Who do you see as your main customers? Will they be self-financing or be mainly paid for by social security or after April 1993 by the local authority? (For more about this, see the 'Introduction', p 13.) What proportion of frail and reasonably fit people will you be looking for? Is there any condition you would not be prepared to care for?

You should think out all these factors clearly when drawing up a contract which you and a potential resident will enter into. Before someone decides on a particular Home, there are a number of questions which will have to be asked on both sides. You, as the Home owner, will have to assess whether the potential resident will fit in with the others already living in the Home, whether the person will be able to enjoy the facilities and activities you offer, or whether he or she is too frail for your staff to cope with comfortably.

On the other hand, you should be prepared for a barrage of questions from the potential resident and his or her relatives. Encourage questions if none are forthcoming. The more you know about each other before any decisions are taken, the less likely you are to encounter problems in the future.

Make clear to the potential resident what they can expect of you and what you expect from them. For instance, it is wise, as mentioned in 'Spotlight on the Residents', to have a trial period, which can be terminated by either party, before any contracts are signed.

The person has the right to know exactly what is included in the fees you are asking, and what constitutes 'extras'. You may have decided that all accommodation, meals, laundry and newspapers are included, whilst items such as dry cleaning, professional hairdressing and specialist fee paying services such as chiropody are to be treated as extras.

The other important points to be covered in the resident's contract include procedures about:
- the care to be provided in the Home;
- the termination of care or for a change of contract;
- residents' complaints;
- special situations such as the death of the resident or a change of ownership of the Home.

A properly worded contract between the Home and each resident will lay down clearly and for everyone to see the conditions under which you have both entered the agreement.

Financial implications

Your choice of resident and the services you offer have financial implications, so you should look very carefully at all the potential needs of your clients for special care and equipment and more staff on duty. What revenue do you need to cover your costs and make a profit? Your choice of clientele may determine how much revenue you will receive especially after April 1993. If you decide on a mix of residents, the local authority grant may fall short of the amount necessary to cover the services you intend to provide to other residents. How will you manage the shortfall?

Do you propose in the future to tender for local authority care contracts? What will it cost you to submit an appropriate tender? Your obligations should be set out clearly in negotiated contracts with all parties who pay you for a service or whom you employ. As explained in the 'Introduction', contracts with public and private care purchasers should state in detail what the care is, how it will be provided and how it will be monitored.

The interior of the Home

As a perspective owner/manager, you will need to consider carefully the structural aspects of the Home to meet residents' needs. The advice of an experienced architect who has worked on similar projects, which you have seen and approved, will be of great value. Keep in touch with your local registration officer, and consult the primary health care team for their advice.

Fixed equipment should be planned when the property is being converted. This includes accessible toilets, bathroom and wall rails, ramps, stair lifts, etc. There are also a number of essential moveable aids. Some of these may be expensive, but there are often alternatives which may be equally effective. It is important to discuss special equipment with other Home owners and to obtain professional advice from a doctor, a physiotherapist or, an occupational therapist about what is and is not necessary. Some essential items of equipment are:

- mobility aids: wheelchairs, frames and walking sticks;
- continence aids: sheets, blankets, commodes, bedpans and urinals;
- lifting equipment for use in baths and beds.

Decoration and colour schemes

Age does not mean that people respond less to colours – Picasso's paintings at eighty were full of vibrancy and colour. If someone has weak eyesight, colour is in fact more important. There has been a lot of research recently into the types of colour to stimulate moods and activity – pale, clear blues and greens provide a relaxing, stimulating atmosphere; yellows are cheerful, and a place with touches of bright red encourages activity.

Furniture and furnishings

The manner in which you furnish the Home will set the atmosphere. Your choices will be partly governed by what your residents need. This includes chairs that they can get easily in and out of, tables where they can put their belongings, beds that are the correct height from the floor and so on. All furniture and furnishings must comply with fire regulations. Some Homes aim for the kind of furnishings that their residents will feel comfortable with, but this has to be tempered by their budget.

Nevertheless, it is possible to provide a homely atmosphere without great cost, with a little imagination and thought. So many Homes have excellent care, but they feel like an institution when you go into them. Others have dingy colours which lower rather than lift the spirits. It is generally agreed that the more a resident feels at home in their room, the better they will settle in. And at any time of life, one of the most crucial ways of feeling at home is to have some of your own things around you.

Owner 'I'm not fussed whether they bring furniture, but I do like them to bring loads of pictures and photographs, things that were their treasures, ornaments. Everybody has something personal that they like very much. It might be a desk or a teddy bear. And I've got one who has a lovely doll, it's a home-made doll and it's really elegantly dressed, it's got all sorts of underwear and things like this.'

Gardens

A garden which is a pleasure to look at and be in will enhance the value of your Home in every way. Trees, shrubs and plants all add to a sense of well-being. Take time to consider the views from the windows, make sure that there is proper access for wheelchairs or people who use sticks or frames.

The average long-term resident will be with you for four years. It is worth while taking the trouble to personalise that stay. For most, it will be the last home they have.

KEY POINTS

- Get professional advice about which items of special equipment are essential.
- The atmosphere of a Home is set off by its colour schemes and the variety of furnishings.
- Allow space for residents' own belongings both in their own rooms and in communal spaces.

RECRUITING STAFF

Good staff are crucial to the successful running of any Home, and this means people who are confident in what they are doing, are able to understand priorities, have a genuinely caring attitude and an understanding of older people. Today, many people have taken a social care training course at a college of further education. This can be added to by being assessed for National Vocational Qualifications (NVQs) at the place of work. Professional care is becoming just that – more professional – and many carers now look for a career structure where they would move on to a Senior Care Assistant grade.

Your staffing needs

Staffing levels have to be matched closely to the aims of a residential home, the numbers of residents and the type of care which is best suited for them.

Almost all Homes will have the following categories of staff: management, administration, personal care, catering and domestic work. Larger establishments may also employ staff to help with training, activities, gardening, etc.

As an ideal, each time a new resident is admitted, the management of a Home should check that there are enough staff in service to provide the type of care and support outlined in each resident's care plan – for instance, help with getting out of bed and with using the toilet, continence management, frequent checks on their whereabouts because of confusion, and so on.

If you are setting up a Home, this kind of assessment will be difficult because you are unlikely to have details about the level of residents' dependency. You should allow for your staffing levels to be flexible during the first few months, possibly by using temporary help, and paying these staff members on an hourly basis. Under these circumstances they can put in more hours if the need arises, and this trial period will allow you to get a feel for future demand without committing yourself to large overheads in the first instance.

NOTE   Any form of special care should be of the type that can be given by a caring friend or relative in their home. Otherwise any nursing required should be provided by a district or community nurse.

In considering the needs of residents in the Home, you will also have to know which of the needs have to be dealt with round the clock by core staff and which can or should be dealt with by people outside. Your Home may have access to community services of the type used by older people with similar requirements who live in their own homes.

Which of the following skill areas do you require from your staff team: at all times (1), regularly (2), occasionally (3)?

Practical tasks

Cleaning	Household maintenance
Cooking	Gardening
Laundry	

Care tasks

Care for residents' possessions

Personal care

Special care, including
administration of drugs

Keywork and emotional care

Group work

Meeting with residents' families

Preparation of reports and records

Counselling

Health care

Medical support

Nursing support

Physiotherapy

Occupational therapy

Dental care

Chiropody

Nutritional advice

Speech therapy

Sight and hearing therapy

Activities

Leisure activities

Creative activities

Exercise classes

Outings and holidays

Managerial and support tasks

Staff management

Household management

Administration

Staff supervision, counselling and training

Do you have a mechanism for making sure that the changing needs of individual residents can be met through modifications to your staffing?

Staffing levels

The Wagner Report recommended that residents should not live in groups of more than 16, and fewer if possible. The idea of small group living is still being debated. Managers who have tried small groups stress that they must be organised sensitively and allow for flexibility – a resident who does not like the group she or he has been assigned to should be able to move to another one. The ideal would be for 40 people in a Home to be divided into 4 groups of 10. This would give them continuity of care by a small team of staff. It should also provide them with a 'family' unit of their own peers.

For example, the sample chart on page 40 shows that 10 residents would need the following staffing levels: a minimum of 2 day-staff on day duty, except after lunch from 2.00–4.00 pm; 1 night-staff member on duty from 10.00 pm–7.00 am; 1 senior member of staff on call at night and 2 available during office hours.

In order to cover holidays, daytime shifts and other time off, it has been estimated that in practice, the cover for day-staff at the above level is the equivalent of 3.6 full-time staff, assuming a 39-hour week. The cover for night time work is estimated at the equivalent of 2.2 full-time staff for a 10-hour period, including sleeping in on call.

These staffing levels should be considered a minimum, and many inspection officers would require higher ones. In a recent survey, most Home owners said that their registration authority required them to have waking staff on duty, as well as someone on call. You should discuss your proposed staffing levels with the local inspectorate at an early stage in your planning.

Managers can also increase staffing levels by offering on-the-job training experience to people on local training schemes.

Appointing staff

In the early days you will probably have to advertise for staff. Even though vacancies are often filled by word of mouth, you should be aware of equal opportunities legislation which advocates that all posts should be fairly advertised. It is essential that you take up references for new staff, even if they are personally known to you. They should also sign the Rehabilitation of Offenders Act declaration.

When you appoint new staff, you have to make a number of decisions and assumptions. You look at qualifications, personal qualities, potential for development and personality. You also attempt to decide if that person will fit in as part of the team already there. Once they are in the post, you need to make sure that you and your senior staff give them advice and support. This may be easy in a small Home, but in some of the large local authority homes a new assistant may feel excluded from a cosy clique that has developed.

You may need to give additional support to a new care assistant from an ethnic minority group who may face racial prejudice from other members of

Sample chart

Suggested staffing levels for a home

NO OF RESIDENTS – 10

CLIENT GROUP – average levels of dependency

TIME	NEEDS	DAY STAFF	NIGHT STAFF	SENIOR COVER
0 Mid-night	Decline in demand.	–	–	1
1	Night staff can do	–	–	1
2	some ancillary work.	–	–	1 sleeping in on call
3		–	–	1
4		–	–	1
5		–	–	1
6		–	–	1
7		–	–	1
8	Heavy period of work.	2	1	1
9	Residents getting up	2	–	2 on duty
10	and breakfasting.	2	–	2
11	General duties in the unit or outside.	2	–	2
12 Noon	Lunch – a peak in	2	–	2
1	demand.	2	–	2
2		2	–	2
3	Slight decline in demand.	1	–	2
4	Tea time – peak in	2	–	2
5	demand.	5	–	1 on duty
6		2	–	1
7	Supper	2	–	1
8	Steady amount of work.	2	–	1
9	Getting residents ready	2	–	1
10	for bed.	–	1	1
11		–	1	1 sleeping in on call
12 Mid-night		–	1	1

staff or from residents. It is part of management's job to notice if this has happened and to take steps to integrate the new assistant.

Staff contracts

All staff should be offered a written contract to include a job description, rates of pay, duties, hours worked, payments for overtime and procedures for dismissal or termination of employment on both sides including the period of notice. All new members of staff, even if they are experienced carers, should also have an induction course to make sure they understand the needs of your Home and its philosophy.

Senior staff

Senior staff in a Home need the same qualities as in any other organisation – leadership qualities, the ability to administer and work with a team, to facilitate care, a mature outlook, the ability to make decisions and to deputise for managers in their absence. In addition, they will need specific skills in all aspects of giving care, including first aid, some understanding of the physiology and psychology of ageing, special care medication, and a good supply of common sense. Above all, they need the ability to respond to residents as people.

Senior staff should also have the ability to build up a good staff team and be able to nurture the people within it. In addition they should be able to manage staff meetings and contribute to training within the Home.

Senior staff should be actively encouraged to attend management training courses, where people are shown examples of good management and asked to examine their own strengths and weaknesses. This way your senior staff become more confident in themselves and also feel a greater sense of your confidence in them. There will be a constant flow of new ideas to be considered and either adopted or rejected, and the stimulus of meeting and mixing with members of staff from other Homes will broaden the outlook of your senior staff.

The reputation of your Home will depend greatly on your choice of staff for senior positions. Their example will be followed by junior members of staff, and their attitude to the residents will be echoed by those who work under them. Whilst the qualities outlined above are important when choosing senior staff, seemingly small matters like good time-keeping, cheerfulness under trying conditions, a sympathetic approach to residents and junior staff and a general air of 'approachability'.

Manager 'I look for someone who has the capacity to analyse and look at a situation and consider that there might be more than one way of solving it.'

Interviewing new staff

Managers should involve their assistants or senior staff when they interview new care staff. These are the people who will have to get along with them on a day-to-day basis and will be able to offer a different viewpoint from yours. Residential homes have a mixture of personalities in their staff, just as the residents have – quiet and reflective, cheerful and outgoing. It's the ability to work in a team where there may be all sorts of different skills that is important. What are some other qualities?

Manager 'I look for the ability to listen, to communicate well. Somebody that has some compassion for the people here, because it's not easy for them, but it's also not easy for care assistants. They should also be quite mature in their attitude, because they come across lots of difficult and distressing situations. It's useful if they are good with their hands, and I believe that common sense and a sense of humour are essential!'

Owner 'When I hire my staff, they seem to be much more mature than I was at that age. I don't think anyone goes into this sort of life without knowing that's what they want. You find some young girls tell me they couldn't bear to work in a shop.

'And it's good career-wise now, they can really do so well. I give them the opportunity of doing a course, if they've been with me for a little while. I send them on a year's day-release to the college because I think the job needs people who have had just that extra bit of training that we can't do here.'

Manager 'On the practical side, I often give people a scenario about Mrs Jones who is frightened of going up in the lift. What sort of things could you dream up on the spot to help her either overcome that fear or get her up the stairs. In most of the solutions to problems in looking after people in Homes there are no right and wrong answers, it's whatever you dream up that works for the staff and that resident. Then I also ask questions like how they would make a new resident feel at home.'

Catering and domestic staff

Often the most important of these, from the point of view of the residents, is the cook or chef, because meals can be the highlight of the day for most people.

Cooking is a difficult job because it is not just the preparation of food and organising the kitchens to cater for twenty or thirty people, it is a major budgeting exercise. There are lots of proprietors who end up doing the cooking themselves because there are so many decisions to be made about what usually appears to be simple. So, in appointing a cook, you will need to look not just for cooking experience for a large number of people but for someone who is able to balance what the residents most enjoy eating with what is nutritionally good for them (see pages 124–125) and what the budget will stand. There will always be people who are on a special diet to be catered for when the cook is planning menus.

Good domestic staff are essential, but not always easy to come by. This is something that you should always check when deciding where to set up a Home. In some private homes, the domestic work is shared by the care staff; in others, contract staff are brought in. What a new owner decides to do will depend very much on the neighbourhood.

Office administrator

Even if you don't require their services for long, it can be very helpful if you bring in an experienced office administrator for the crucial early days when you may have to run around making sure everything else is going smoothly. She or he can set up a filing system, rota sheets, holiday lists and the accounts. Some Homes now have their accounts and some of their residents' records on computer. This is something you may like to consider. A good filing system will include personal and confidential files for staff and residents, as discussed in more detail on page 112.

KEY POINTS

- Senior staff represent you in your absence, so they should understand your aims and objectives.

- Senior staff need to be able to relate to all visitors coming into the Home. Good links with the community are vitally important to the well-being of residents.

- Many care staff look for a career progression and expect to get training while they are employed.

- When appointing care staff, look for people who can work in a team, who genuinely like older people and are concerned to give time to them when necessary.

- A good cook is an important ingredient in a good Home.

Spotlight on the Residents

This chapter looks at what it is like being in a Home from the residents' point of view as individuals whose first need is to be treated as a person.

May 'You have to learn to be middle-aged and old aged. I found it very difficult at first because I can't do all the things I used to do, I have to rely on other people, which made me very frustrated – people wouldn't bring me the right things, or they cooked in a different way. But it's no good being negative about it, you must just realise that bit by bit you will get used to it.'

Men and women who are now in their eighties and nineties, those like May quoted above, were born when horse-drawn vehicles had to make way for motor cars on our roads, when Germany was ruled by the Kaiser, when aeroplanes had not been invented and when telegrams were transmitted by morse code. That generation has had to come to terms with far more changes than anyone born after 1945. They are survivors.

It is also true that this generation has probably known more poverty than any of their grandchildren and great-grandchildren will. By the time wages and conditions of work were rising for the rest of the population in the 60's, most older people were drawing out their small pension and still having to 'make do'.

Now they come to our residential homes. Some of them are frail, some are confused and unhappy. Many feel that they have no purpose in life, that they are useless. But many also find care and a loving environment.

A MOVING-IN PROCEDURE

Often people find the move to a Home one of the most traumatic moments of their lives. Many become withdrawn and acutely depressed, some die within the first few weeks. So it is vitally important for them to have support and loving care during this period. There is not only the trauma of the change of home – one of the highest percentages on the scale of life stress – but also the strangeness of suddenly living in a community which is, for many, the first time in their lives. On the positive side, admission to a Home can be a chance to improve someone's quality of life if they have been in hospital or living alone and finding it harder to cope.

How people are admitted to a residential home depends very much on circumstances. It is best to offer a trial period (usually four to six weeks) to a prospective resident to enable them to get the feel of the Home and to find out whether it provides care suited to their needs. One Home carries out a procedure outlined below, which has proved very successful.

Before the resident arrives

Care staff are told something about the new resident, and one of them usually accompanies the manager on a home visit. They explain what will happen on the day of admission and also suggest that the person might like to bring some furniture or personal possessions. Any friends or relatives present are given a warm invitation to come to the Home as often as they like, and as soon as possible. Finally, a date is arranged for the new resident to come and visit the Home before the final admission.

During this period, the manager will also make contact with social workers if they have been concerned with the admission, so that the care staff can find out any relevant information about the person.

The first few days

If there are no relatives to help, the same care assistant goes to the person's home, checks that he or she has everything, and takes them personally to the residential home.

On arrival, the new resident is given some tea and biscuits in her room while her things are brought up, and then the care assistant helps her unpack. Some people prefer not to go to the lounge or dining room on their first day, and their wishes are respected – a tray is sent up. If they want to join in, the care assistant shows them round the Home and introduces them to other residents.

In the next few days, all the care staff come and introduce themselves to the new arrival, and try to help them begin to feel at home. Going somewhere new can be frightening at any age. As people get older, fear and loneliness may be very great. This early period is often seen as provisional on both sides, so that a resident has the chance to move if the Home is just not right. The manager also arranges and expects social work support during this trial period.

Staff will need to monitor each new resident very closely – their emotional needs, mental and physical disabilities – and discuss assessment and making up a care plan. They introduce the new resident to any volunteer visitors, and encourage relatives to come to the Home as much as they can. The trial period when a new resident as well as the staff and manager have a chance to see whether 'the shoe fits' should be followed by a review session where everyone involved with that resident – and the resident – can express all their reservations about the Home and hopefully its good points.

Assessment after admission

During the first month to six weeks, the new resident is involved in an assessment of all his or her conditions and needs. This is one of the keys to that person's future in the Home. It may include their reaction to coming into the Home, their general mental and emotional state down to basic things like sleep pattern, continence, speech, dental problems, how good their hearing is and so on. A manager will keep records of all discussions with the resident and any other people involved in the admission, including relatives, so that a proper plan of care can be drawn up. For assessment of people by local authorities after April 1993, see 'Introduction', page 14.

A case conference

In many Homes there is also a meeting or case conference which is attended by the resident, and a member of his or her family if they wish this, a senior staff member of the Home, a district nurse, perhaps a physiotherapist or occupational therapist and a social worker who might be from a community team or attached to the residential home. The meeting gives everyone who has been in contact with the client a chance to pool their knowledge and explore various courses of action. This is not always easy, as different professions have different terms of reference and jargon.

The following guidelines for a case conference have been suggested by the Social Care Association.

– Appoint a neutral chairperson to mediate between different disciplines and act as advocate for the resident.

– The chairperson should make sure that all issues are discussed with sensitivity to the resident's feelings.

– Each participant should come prepared to offer analysis of the resident's needs and a suitable course of action. This of course should include the resident.

– One person should act as secretary to take detailed notes of the meeting, with a summary of all recommendations, to be circulated within two weeks.

– A typical agenda for the meeting could be: identifying needs, making plans, deciding how these should be monitored and reviewed.

Making a care plan

The kind of care discussed will naturally vary with different people. One resident may be physically active but suffer from confusion or depression, another may have a leg ulcer which is very painful and needs a management routine supervised by a district nurse, a third may be very arthritic and would benefit chiefly from exercise and physiotherapy.

After the meeting, the final care plan is agreed with the resident and sent to all concerned with carrying out the recommendations, who may not necessarily have been at the meeting. The care plan usually includes: a summary of the residents physical and emotional needs; his or her contacts outside the Home; the professional carers' recommendations for the treatment of the person's physical and mental conditions.

Two other points not often discussed are on the checklist of some primary health care teams. These are the resident's sexual responses (see page 55) and their fears of dying and death (see page 127).

All residents' care plans should be monitored regularly and updated. This should be a part of regular office routine in a bring-forward file.

KEY POINTS

- Make the admission procedure as gentle as possible – it can be an traumatic experience.

- Arrange for early assessment of a new resident's needs and make sure a care plan is drawn up.

- Make sure any recommendations are acted on and kept on file.

THE RESIDENTS' RIGHTS

At this stage, the new resident becomes part of the Home. It is now their home and as such should be a place where they feel at home. Residents pay for their care from income and savings and are sometimes entitled to State benefits to help with the fees. After April 1993, new residents needing financial support will be paid for as outlined in the 'Introduction', page 13.

Older people sometimes don't like claiming social security benefits, but they have probably contributed to central and local government funds through paying rates, the community charge and income tax. Residents have the right to expect good care, and managers and owners have obligations to them. The resident's rights will usually include:

–   being able to live a fulfilling life;

–   to be treated with dignity as an individual;

–   to have personal privacy for themselves and their affairs;

–   to do things at their own pace and when they want to do them;

–   to be consulted and involved in their personal care;

–   to have their cultural, sexual and religious needs respected;

–   to associate with whom they wish;

–   to keep up contacts within the community;

–   to have access to community services and facilities;

- to perform any activity they feel capable of doing;
- not to be forced to do anything against their will;
- to take any risks implied by these rights without being unnecessarily restricted.

Some of these rights are mentioned elsewhere in the book, and many are matters of common sense. They are closely related to the basic human needs experienced by all of us for a comfortable living and working environment, a sense of security, of belonging and being loved, of being respected as a person, of having a sense of purpose in life.

Residential homes are able to meet basic human needs to some degree, but doing so makes demands on management and staff. In Homes where the aim is to give people what they need, ideas are constantly being discussed and questioned informally and in formal staff meetings. Individual needs are all relevant from the moment when a resident takes the decision to enter a Home. It can be hard sometimes for a younger generation to understand the feelings and needs of someone who is very old – not to lump them all together to be washed, dressed, sat in front of the television, taken to the toilet, fed and put to bed. It leaves out the individual.

Resident 'Caring means treating you as a human being. Very often people look old, they look like a cabbage. But you are always more aware than people think you are.'

Doing things at their own pace

There are very few generalisations one can make about older people, but almost without exception they hate to be rushed. Everything takes just that little bit longer, and they need to be given time to do it. Otherwise, the person may get flustered, upset, trip over something, feel unhappy and guilty about causing trouble and so on.

The right to privacy

One of the most common complaints about residential homes for older people is lack of privacy, in particular where people have to share rooms. Sometimes the beds are in separate areas and screened from each other. But often they are only a couple of feet apart.

In Autumn 1990, the organisation Council and Care visited 84 residential and 30 Homes with dual registration to assess the quality of privacy. These were some of their findings:

- In over 80 per cent of the Homes residents had to share a room.
- 70 per cent of Homes expected residents to use commodes within the hearing of their room-mates.
- In 14 per cent of Homes there was no lockable lavatory.
- In more than half the Homes it was impossible for residents to lock the doors to their rooms.
- In some Homes residents were expected to carry out basic bodily functions in public view, where commodes or wash basins were unscreened.

These facts offend the most basic right to privacy. In general, poorer residents and those who were reliant on social security benefits, suffered disproportionately, often being priced out of private space.

Former manager 'If I could do anything, the first thing I would do is get rid of the double rooms. They're not good news because there's no privacy. People have different times for doing things – different times for going to bed. Using a commode is not pleasant if someone else is in the room.'

If a manager is appointed to a Home where such lack of privacy is common practice, it may not be possible to stop sharing, but provision of screens or room dividers should be a first essential. The ideal would be to give people single rooms if they so wish. Every resident should also be provided with a lockable cupboard or locker for their private possessions.

Residents' financial affairs

It is very important that people do not feel they have lost control of their own affairs once they move into a residential Home, and this is an area which may require tact and sensitivity. Paul Brearley in his book *Working in Residential Homes for Elderly People* points out that staff in a Home should be guided by the principle that they are there to enable residents to do what they cannot do for themselves. This applies to spending their money as much as to helping them take a bath or going out with them to the shops.

In its section on residents' finances, *Home Life* reminds managers that the choice of what residents do with their money is their own. In local authority homes, the authority collects benefits for all their residents in bulk. These residents and those in the private or voluntary sector who are sponsored by local authorities or the DSS, have a weekly cash allowance built into their benefits which managers should make freely available. Non-sponsored residents in a private or voluntary Home normally look after their own finances – they keep their pension book, collect their pension and benefits, tie that up with any other income and pay their bills.

All private and voluntary Homes should have a clearly laid down policy which guarantees residents complete freedom in their financial affairs and access to their money at all times, including petty cash to pay for small daily purchases. Regular payments or fees may be arranged through a bank or building society standing order. This is best sorted out when a resident comes into the Home. Any person who wishes to put some of their money into a bank or another kind of savings account should be enabled to do so.

You can assist residents in handling their affairs by making sure that a list of all charges for services is on display and has been clearly set out in contracts with residents. This gives them the opportunity to raise queries or complaints if they are dissatisfied. You should also give each resident a monthly receipt stating what charges have been made and for which items.

Wills and gifts

All residents should be encouraged to make a Will, with the advice if necessary from the Citizen's Advice Bureau or an independent solicitor and not someone attached to the Home. Members of staff should not witness a Will except in an extreme emergency, and in no circumstances should a member of staff or Home owner/manager become an executor of a Will.

There should also be a clear policy that staff members, which includes the owner, should not accept gifts or tips from residents, except for small token presents. Often this is covered in the staff contract.

Enduring Power of Attorney

There are no fixed guidelines on handling residents' financial affairs when they become too disabled, ill or confused to do this themselves, except for the recommendation that Home managers or owners should not take on this responsibility.

Social services team leader 'From time to time, Home owners have also taken responsibility for managing a resident's financial matters, but there is a conflict of interests and it does leave them in a difficult position. In my view it is best for the resident to have someone from outside the Home who can take on this role, and to some extent act as an advocate.'

Older people can appoint someone who they can trust to look after their affairs if they are capable of understanding the nature of the power which is being granted. If they create an Enduring Power of Attorney (EPA) they can arrange that the power continues if they become mentally incapable. If this does happen, the person named as the Attorney has to apply for the Enduring Power to be registered at the Court of Protection (see p 166).

If a resident is already incapable of appointing an Attorney and their only income is from the state, application can be made to the Department of Social Security for their benefits to be managed by an Appointee. Otherwise it may be necessary to apply to the Court of Protection for the appointment of a Receiver to handle their affairs. Attorneys, Appointees and Receivers may be a relative or friend, solicitor or other suitable person. Some residents' financial affairs may be looked after by someone appointed by social services or a voluntary group such as Age Concern.

NOTE   For information about how the law applies in Scotland you should contact Scottish Action on Dementia at the address on page 167.

Taking risks

There are a number of areas where a manager needs to allow residents to take risks and to have responsibility for his or her actions. For example, allowing people to go out to the shops if they want to, encouraging them to use sticks rather than a wheelchair can be positive provided these 'risks' are carefully calculated and discreetly monitored. Allowing residents to behave responsibly regarding their medication can also give them a sense of self-reliance. Again, tactful checking may be necessary, but the resident's feeling of self-worth will be enhanced. This might mean that a person gets lost, has a fall or perhaps forgets to take prescribed drugs at the correct time, but there are many men and women in their nineties who manage to be self-reliant in those matters without accident.

Psychologist 'Just as we allow small children to take risks in order to develop their independence, so we need to allow their great-grandparents to take risks in order to maintain theirs.'

Care assistant 'There's a kitchen in our unit and we encourage residents to help themselves, make tea and so on. Someone may leave a tap on, or find it hard to lift a kettle, but I believe it's up to them to do it if they want to.'

Being valued

Many older people say that one of the hardest things to bear in old age is the feeling that you are no longer of use to anyone. But even at the point of death, men and women can give support to those who are apparently supporting them. However frail a person is mentally, you can still give them a sense of their own value by talking to them as an equal and by listening to what they say.

Care assistant 'Even though they're talking to you and it might not sound sensible, you respond and help them to have a conversation. And we're learning as well because most the them talk about past experiences before we were even born. So at the same time as giving them conversation, they're helping us. And by meeting their needs, they know that we care.'

Involve the residents

Where possible, residents should be involved in their own care plan and invited to contribute to the running of the Home. This may occur through informal liaison between staff and residents or in a more formal way through a residents' committee, which will be covered in more detail in a later chapter.

Owner 'I've had residents help prepare meals, take the dog for a walk, take responsibility for the flowers if they've been keen gardeners. If they're able, I encourage everything that makes them feel part of the Home. You have to remember it is their home.'

Relative 'My gran was in a Home for three years where the residents helped during mealtimes. Gran's job was to peel the potatoes and she really liked doing it. She wasn't as quick as she was when I first knew her as a child, but no one rushed her. She just took it at her own pace and there was always a lot of noise from the kitchen when it was vegetable peeling time. They seemed to be having a really good time!'

This involvement gives residents the opportunity to work with others on equal terms, it makes them feel needed and it provides simple exercise for mind and hands. However, staff often object because domestic duties are slowed down and extra provision is required, while residents may feel that these tasks are the staff's duties. Involving the residents may require some work towards changing the attitudes of both staff and residents.

The spiritual dimension

Many older people draw comfort and support from religion and welcome visits from someone connected with their particular faith or someone who takes into account more than their daily routine and care. You may need to take time to find out from people of different faiths or ethnic groups in the Home what will bring them the spiritual support they may need.

Owner 'The vicar from across the road, he comes and they have a Communion service. And I take a lot of them out to Church every week, and there's a nun who comes once a week and just sits and talks to them. It's all part of helping to make life worthwhile for them.'

Senior care assistant 'Sometimes I just put on a record, not dance music or anything like that, but something quiet and peaceful, and it just changes the atmosphere. Even Millie who just sits there most of the time, I've seen her nod her head and listen and sometimes a smile comes on her face.'

Emotions and sexuality

Some residents find rewarding friendships in their new home, but managers need to be aware that the expression of sexuality may be an issue for some of their residents. This needs to be dealt with sensitively, with respect for the privacy of those concerned, and if possible identified and aired before it becomes a problem – to carers and other residents, that is. It is not usually a problem for the people concerned.

Sexual feelings are usually part of an emotional link – people can fall in love at any age. Sexuality in old age does not have to be penetrative sex – it may include mutual masturbation. There are many erotic things two people can do which do not involve the 'normal' sex act. And non-sexual activities like listening to music together can also be very erotic as well as expressing emotions. Counsellors believe that for older people it is important to place a value on emotions and loving. For a fuller discussion of sexuality in older people, see *Living, Loving and Ageing* also published by Age Concern England (details on page 176.)

Residents' pets

Many older people have had a pet of their own at home and may be very distressed at having to part with it. They may find a great deal of pleasure in animals around the residential home. These can range from budgies and goldfish to a cat or dog, though clearly a Home owner will have to restrict the number of animals. A cat, which is less boisterous, may be more appropriate in a place where there are many frail elderly people.

The therapeutic value of stroking is now well documented and the company of a pet is soothing, stimulating and gives you something to love. Unlike many care routines, this does not happen at fixed times. Animals have a will of their own and bring an element of pleasant surprise into the life of a Home – curled up in an unexpected spot, complaining because it's dinner time or coming up to someone and asking to be stroked.

Freedom of choice

Many Homes provide a variety of activities, and someone who has spent a lot of time organising these may feel aggrieved if residents don't want to take part. But while some people enjoy them, others feel they are undignified or just don't want to join in. Residents should be able to choose whether to sit in their rooms or stay in the lounge, whether to play bingo or not, when they go to bed and when they get up. On the medical side, all residents have a legal right to choose their own GP.

```
KEY POINTS
```

- Each person is the sum of their whole life, not just of the present, and has needs as a human being.

- Make sure new residents know their rights and what they can expect of a Home.

- The right to privacy is a key right, but one which very many Homes ignore.

- Giving someone choice means the right for them to say 'No'.

- Creating a sense of well-being means taking into account the emotional and spiritual needs of residents.

GETTING TO KNOW A NEW RESIDENT

As a new resident begins to settle into a Home, the process of getting to know each other begins. And like any new encounter, it takes a little time. The care staff will see the person every day, but what of the owner or manager? In a large Home, it can be all too easy for Mr Smith to be a name on a file. In a smaller Home, the owner will probably be involved at a more personal level early on and be able to find out who that person is underneath.

There are often tragedies in someone's life that may explain why that person is the way they are. A child dead, redundancy and a hard life on the dole, a marriage that has gone wrong or the death of a partner after many years, leaving the other alone, bewildered, depressed and neglectful of themselves.

But there are also the high spots – the time when a deal was pulled off and they went home for a holiday in the West Indies, the daughter whose name features in the papers, the friend who gave support when a partnership went wrong.

People reveal themselves if you take the time to sit and talk, ask questions about a photograph or listen in at a reminiscence session. It helps you to see each person in the round, and when you give of your time – quality time – he or she gets to know you as well, and begins to trust you.

Owner 'Most of my residents have lived round here – a lot of people retire to Somerset, so I see their friends as much as their family. Often their family is up near London so they don't come down very often. And it's friends who visit, so I get to know not just Mrs James, but her ex-neighbour, and someone she use to play bridge with, and someone who walks her dog. I try and keep it a family atmosphere as much as possible.'

Living day to day

Once a new resident is settled in, there will be other things to discover and these may form part of a person's care plan and therapy. This is the time to find out what sort of things they enjoy and are still able to do. Even a very frail person can listen to music, watch videos of old films (or new ones) or sit in the garden. If someone can't read, perhaps they could be read to. Encourage the care staff to find out about likes and dislikes as well, what food they enjoy, and what can be done to make the time more agreeable. In so many Homes the television is switched on, the residents sit round it in a circle, and yet no one is watching or listening.

Minority interests

Older people, like the rest of the population, are made up of all kinds of groupings. Some have had families, some are single, most are heterosexual but some are homosexual. They are from different social classes and ethnic groups and they have differing or no religious beliefs.

Every Home will have residents from one or more of these groups, and a person who has chosen to live in a particular Home has the right to have his or her cultural background or beliefs respected. Sometimes you will notice these as soon as a new resident arrives, but sometimes care staff and managers may have to ask questions or talk to their families and friends.

In a Home where there are mixed groupings of residents, certain types of food, and the Home's normal social activities, which may go down well with one set of people may be quite inappropriate for another. Sometimes there are language barriers between staff and residents, and you may need to call in a translator to improve communication about any problems a resident may have or to describe procedures in the Home which may be unfamiliar. Managers need to be sensitive to what is appropriate in these circumstances, and this is an area where special training of staff can be very helpful (see pages 119–120).

Negotiating with residents

Older people are human, and that means that they can be as kind and considerate or as difficult, territorial, demanding and selfish, as the rest of us. There may be good reasons why someone is driving you up the wall. That doesn't make their actions any less irritating. A manager may have to be assertive if a person gets furious when a newcomer is sitting in their chair – either with the established resident, or with the newcomer. Either way, tact and diplomacy will be in order.

Then there are people who have eccentric wants, where some negotiation has to take place.

Owner 'In our Home, one of the elderly gentlemen likes to read in his room till two or three am. So I arranged for the night staff to bring him up tea and biscuits at 2.30 am. Sometimes he likes a chat and sometimes he doesn't. Usually he's then ready to go to bed, and may need some help.'

Allowing friendships to develop

Often residents will find someone in the Home whom they can relate to, and quite deep friendships result. Sometimes, a deep bond can also develop between residents and staff. This can in some cases cause difficulties. Managers should support friendships that develop between residents or residents and staff, unless one side is being exploited – ie it becomes obvious that a 'friendship' between two residents is based on financial grounds only, or the good nature of one of your members of staff is being taken for granted by a particular resident.

In one case reported in the magazine *Care Weekly*, a member of staff arranged for a resident to have a short break by going away with her own family. To her horror, this caused jealousy among other members of staff, and accusations of favouritism. But people within any organisation do develop friendships or deeper relationships. As long as neither side is taking advantage of the other, managers should not allow something that is clearly bringing joy into a resident's life to be crushed.

Dealing with abuse

Any person who is vulnerable may have their situation abused. Abuse of older people does happen in their own homes and in residential homes. Local authorities are developing guidance on the recognition of abuse. Managers should always be aware of the dangers of abuse and take prompt actions to deal with it. There are a number of ways in which an elderly person can be abused by care staff, which may be through physical violence or through psychological or emotional methods.

The signs of physical violence may not be obvious, but they usually include bruising and a history of so-called self-inflicted injuries from falls or clumsiness and reports from members of staff of someone being 'difficult'. Some of the worst forms of psychological abuse have included restraining people to a chair, giving them sedative drugs which they have not been prescribed and tying someone with incontinence to a commode. Less extreme forms of abuse are personal neglect, lack of any mental or physical stimulation, lack of privacy and being deprived of any personal possessions.

A resident who has been physically abused is likely to be nervous when a staff member comes too near, and they may also be prone to depression or to strike out. If you suspect that any of your residents are suffering from any form of abuse, it is essential to call in professional advice, usually from the GP, who may refer the resident to a community psychiatric nurse or the social services department. If the person is able to make a complaint, then the complaints procedure should be followed and the abuser confronted. If the person is confused and unable to complain formally, you should ask a social worker for advice. They may appoint an advocate who will take up the complaint on behalf of the resident.

Is restraint necessary?

Any person who restrains another against their consent has to be able to justify the action in law. Otherwise they can be charged with trespass to the person, assault and battery or false imprisonment. A person's consent may be implied from their conduct and does not necessarily have to be stated.

Problems arise where a resident may not be mentally capable of giving informed consent because they are in a progressive state of confusion or dementia. When there is no consent, restraint may be justified in common law, but managers should refer to chapter 18 of the code of practice of the Mental Health Act, 1983.

This is clearly a difficult area, and if you have residents in your Home where you feel some form of restraint may occasionally be necessary, you should take advice from the GP and the inspection unit and make sure that you and all the staff have the knowledge and training to deal with potentially difficult situations. But your first responsibility as manager is to protect the resident's individual right to freedom of action.

Moving someone on

Occasionally a problem arises when the increasing frailty of a resident becomes too difficult for care staff to handle. In this case, arrangements can be made with the resident or his or her relatives and the GP to transfer to a nursing home where the proper level of nursing care can be given. Sometimes a resident becomes mentally unbalanced and difficult to control. Under these circumstances the resident's GP may refer him or her to a psycho-geriatrician who may recommend transfer either temporarily or permanently into a psychiatric hospital.

Ideally, there should be a stated procedure for dealing with residents who become disruptive. This should involve an independent assessment of the resident's needs and should give the resident and his or her relatives an opportunity to appeal against the assessment.

As mentioned in the chapter 'Branching Out', it is important to keep in touch with other Home owners. You will each have your own special areas of expertise and this could prove extremely helpful to distressed relatives should the occasion arise when you can no longer care for a particular resident. Maybe you know of another Home in the area that caters for the more frail resident. This of course also works in reverse, and perhaps you will be recommended by another Home owner.

KEY POINTS

- Encourage staff to get to know a new resident and spend as much time with him or her as they can.
- People with minority interests or way of life should be able to take a full part in the life of the Home, but to have their dietary needs or

customs respected.

- Keep watch for signs of abuse and take immediate steps to stop it. Staff should know their legal duties as well as residents' rights.

- You may need to refer to a resident's GP in dealing with situations of abuse or when restraint seems necessary.

- Friendships between residents may develop into deeper relationships. Managers should be aware of the danger of exploitation (see page 59).

Health in Old Age

Although all of us grow old, no one dies of old age – and disability and ill health are not inevitable. Many specific illnesses can be treated, and conditions like incontinence can be managed or alleviated to allow sufferers a better quality of life.

The physical and psychological welfare of older people requires a combination of medical and nursing expertise, good personal care from well trained staff in the Home, combined with common sense and an understanding of residents' needs and wishes – and a loving touch.

In this chapter we outline the most common ailments among people of 75 and over: declining mobility, impaired eyesight and hearing and difficulties with the circulatory, respiratory, digestive, glandular, urinary and nervous systems, including depression and dementia. There are practical suggestions for the care or treatment of common illnesses as well as for care of the mouth, leg ulcers, feet and teeth. Those wanting more complete information about health problems not covered may wish to refer to 'Recommended Reading' on page 168.

The chapter also covers the proper handling of residents' medicines and a summary of complementary therapies which are now being used in some hospitals and in the general care of older people.

PHYSICAL CONDITIONS

There are a number of conditions which may affect older people in a residential home. Although they may not be life-threatening, they should be monitored and managed as far as possible to improve the general quality of the resident's life.

Most of the treatment of these conditions (as well as psychological and neurological ones) given under the National Health Service is free, but there are some things for which most people have to pay part or all of the cost. For details about financial help with dental charges, sight tests and glasses, elastic stockings, wigs and fabric supports, you should refer to the book *Your Rights* also published by Age Concern England (details on page 175). In addition there are the free factsheets *Dental Care in Retirement* and *Help with Incontinence* (details on page 178).

Declining mobility

Over 60 per cent of people above the age of 75 are troubled by arthritis or rheumatism, which can range from slight stiffness to considerable pain and difficulty in moving. As we get older, nearly everyone suffers from osteoarthrosis (also called osteoarthritis or OA) to some extent: general wear and tear leads to some degeneration of the joints, especially those of the legs and spine. Allied to this is unsteadiness on the feet which has many causes. Among these are: the ageing of the mechanism of balance, unsuitable medicines, heart disease or the after-effects of a stroke.

Aids and equipment

Many elderly people use sticks, walking frames or wheelchairs to help themselves keep mobile and improve their stability. An outdoor wheelchair which a staff member or another resident can push will do much to improve the quality of life for someone with poor walking ability. There are other types of chair which can be pushed by a disabled resident or operated electrically.

Any resident who may be in need of a wheelchair should have a skilled assessment of their needs, since wheelchairs are often prescribed inappropriately. In some health authorities this assessment is carried out by the community occupational therapy department, in others it is the responsibility of a physiotherapist. Residents should be discouraged from buying a wheelchair from a mail order catalogue. If they want to try one out it should be done at a disabled living centre, as part of the assessment. For the address of a centre near the Home, contact RADAR at the address on page 167.

Wheelchairs can be obtained on free long-term loan through disablement service centres or the local health authority's medical loans department, with a doctor's signature on the application. Short-term loans can be arranged through the Red Cross or other voluntary organisations.

When a resident is admitted to the Home, you should make sure that any special equipment which they require, such as lifting devices or special baths, is installed and ready for use.

Aids for daily living such as special cutlery and dressing aids can be bought from specialist outlets or by mail order. You can get information about the range of available aids from the Disabled Living Foundation at the address on page 166. Occupational therapists can offer suggestions about improvising aids for people with mobility difficulties which are often as effective as those from a specialist firm, at a fraction of the cost.

Help with mobility problems

There is no known cure for rheumatoid or osteoarthritis, but there is much which can be done to make them easier to live with. Operations for hip replacement joints are safe and common, although there may be a long waiting list for hospital admission. Sufferers of both types of arthritis may be prescribed analgesics, anti-inflammatory agents or other medicines to reduce pain and inflammation.

Many older people are in the habit of buying their own medication. They may benefit from recent research which has shown that paracetamol is as effective in relieving arthritic conditions as aspirin or ibuprofen and related drugs but does not cause gastric bleeding or other intestinal side effects. Paracetamol is dangerous in overdose, and as with all medicines must be kept secure from children visiting the Home.

For milder cases of osteoarthritis, specific exercises, movement and physiotherapy are the most important methods of keeping stiffness at bay, although they may be unlikely to alter the course of the disease. Warmth from an electrically heated pad may also be comforting. Recent research has shown that people with an average age of 80 have been able to gain significant mobility with the help of regular physiotherapy combined with improved footwear and walking aids. The less people use their limbs, the less mobile they become – the 'if you don't use it you lose it' syndrome. For ways of managing pain, see page 83.

Regular exercise is one of the most important things a good Home can offer in maintaining the health and mobility of its residents. Make sure each resident has a care plan which includes advice on exercise and mobility as appropriate. You should also ensure that relatives and friends understand the plan as well. Encourage all residents to walk when they are able, even if it takes longer, rather than go in a wheelchair. Many people often don't feel inclined to walk for its own sake, but may be willing to walk to the dining room with a little encouragement.

Provide formal and informal occasions when residents can have the opportunity to move or exercise – anything from old time dancing to a straight exercise session with one of the care staff. There are excellent booklets and tapes produced by the organisation EXTEND which can be used with individuals or groups (see address on page 166).

Problems with falling

There are many different causes of falls. Some can be prevented – for instance, you should keep a look-out for obvious hazards which someone can trip over. Try to keep small pieces of furniture, personal belongings, electrical leads and walking sticks or frames away from passageways where people walk.

Rooms and public places should be well lit, although the lights should not be too glaring as this can actually worsen the eyesight of someone with a cataract. As people age, their ability to see in the dark halves every seven years, so they rely on good lighting to see where they are going. All Homes should have some provision for emergency lighting and also heating.

Make sure that places with a change of level such as stairs and steps are well-lighted and are clearly marked and have a rail which continues for a few metres beyond the top and bottom of the stairs.

Encourage staff to be on the look-out for handbags, sticks or frames, which could cause people to trip and fall. Check for rugs or lino with curling edges. Make sure that all residents who are known to be unsteady have suitable walking aids. A good rule of thumb is that residents who fall twice within a year should have a thorough medical check with a careful review of their medicines.

Impaired eyesight and hearing

Poor eyesight and being hard of hearing are problems for around 40 per cent of the population over 75 – and for those in residential homes, with a higher average age, the figure is likely to be greater. Both disabilities lead to poor communication with staff and other residents, and also cut residents off from television and the radio.

Managing these conditions

The first step is to encourage anyone who you think has a problem with their eyesight or is having difficulty hearing to have a thorough assessment of their condition. If they have never worn spectacles before or particularly a hearing aid, they may need some help and support in learning to use them.

When a person with poor eyesight enters the Home, encourage them to register as partially sighted or blind with the local hospital eye clinic. They are then able to borrow special low vision aids from the hospital eye service. Such aids are also provided for a fee by a charity, the Partially Sighted Society. A resident with hearing difficulties may be referred by their GP for tests at a local hospital.

Staff should be trained to approach residents with sight or hearing difficulties in a gentle manner, perhaps with a slight touch to indicate their presence. It is important that their presence is recognised before they speak, and they should tell residents with poor sight when they are leaving the room. Staff should speak slowly and distinctly and look at the person, with their face clearly visible.

Staff should also be aware of the tendency most people have of shouting at a deaf person and you should make sure they do not do this. The best way of talking to a deaf person is to lower your voice in pitch, as they can't hear high tones, to speak slowly with gestures and to use phrases which suggest the same message in a different way, such as "Would you like to go to lunch now, because it's one o'clock and it's time for us to eat?" This gives the deaf person several different pointers as to what is being said.

For residents with sight problems, books on cassette provide entertainment and stimulation, and you should contact the Royal National Institute for the Blind about its Talking Book Service. A changing selection of large-type books may be arranged through your local library. Reading matter and tapes may also be provided through local voluntary organisations. For special appliances adapted for residents who are hard of hearing or with sight problems, you may want to contact reputable local stores about telephones with large numerals or a TV with a teletext facility. The Royal National Institute for the Deaf has information about the induction loop system. Addresses of all these organisations are on pages 166–167.

One of the banes of many residential homes is the constant noise of the television, often set within a circle of people sitting passively round – few actually watching. A recent development, which Home managers may find useful, is an audio transmitter attached to the television. It relays the sound to individual headphones, amplifying it if necessary. The device has the double advantage of silencing the insistent television sound, (which may encourage conversation), and as everyone can wear headphones, a deaf person is not marked out from the rest.

Hearing aids

Hearing aids and batteries are available on free loan from a local NHS hearing centre, or they may be bought privately. These are usually expensive, though they may have extras such as a remote control which makes turning the volume up or down easier. Some advertisements make great claims for deaf aids, and a resident should always be encouraged to get one for a trial period before parting with any money.

Hearing aids are not of course a cure-all for someone with hearing problems. The human ear selects the sounds it wants to hear, but a hearing aid has no such discrimination. This means that there may be a constant wash of sound in the ear, which may cause not just annoyance but also confusion, especially in a large room with a lot of noise going on. People with aids often choose to switch them off part of the time. If a resident is having difficulty adjusting to using an aid, get in touch with the British Association for the Hard of Hearing, which has a network of local advisers.

Heart disease

Heart trouble, including angina, and heart irregularities affect over a quarter of the elderly population. The most serious form is coronary thrombosis, when a clot of blood forms in the coronary artery taking blood to the heart and causes a stoppage in the blood supply. A large blockage will cause death. A smaller thrombosis will usually cause the victim to collapse with sudden, severe pain in the centre of the chest which sometimes radiates into the neck or arms. You should seek medical treatment urgently and sit the person in a comfortable, fairly upright position such as in an armchair, loosen their clothing and give assurance that help is coming. Sometimes older people suffer a coronary attack without severe pain, and the condition is only picked up through an electrocardiograph (ECG).

At least two or three months' convalescence is needed after a heart attack so that the scar tissue can form and smaller blood vessels can take over from the damaged artery. Very gentle progressive exercise is usually prescribed during the convalescence period.

Other heart conditions include heart failure, which often occurs at night accompanied by a feeling of breathlessness and a feeling of drowning. Again, emergency treatment is essential and the person should be made comfortable by sitting up with their legs hanging over the edge of a bed or chair.

Angina is a chest pain due to an inadequate blood supply to the heart, often caused by hardened arteries. The pain may be brought on by cold, emotion, exercise or exertion. Common symptoms of heart trouble are swelling of ankles and breathlessness, particularly during the night, though all of these may be due to other conditions needing different treatment. A resident who has any of these symptoms of any severity should have a medical assessment.

Management

Those residents who are able should take some form of exercise (within the limits of their pain or breathlessness) which will stimulate the circulation and strengthen the heart muscle. This should be carried out under the guidance of the GP.

A variety of medicines are often prescribed for heart conditions. On no account should care staff take it upon themselves to adjust a resident's dosage without consulting their doctor. Staff may also need to check, tactfully, that someone does not get in the habit of altering their own dosage. Older people often tend to alter their diuretic tablets if they find the effects uncomfortable or annoying, but any alteration can lead to serious complications.

One exception to this is glycerol trinitrate, which is prescribed for the specific relief of angina and where the person may vary the dose according to the severity of the pain.

Respiration

Some residents may suffer from breathlessness because of heart failure, or a chest disease such as bronchitis, emphysema or asthma. Proper diagnosis is essential for effective treatment. If a resident has a cold and begins to cough up yellow sputum, this usually means that the cold has developed into bronchitis, then the resident may develop other symptoms such as shortness of breath. If a resident develops a chest infection, you should call a doctor, who may prescribe drugs. Physiotherapy and gentle exercise may help a sufferer's chest to move more freely and make the best use of lung power.

Influenza is another illness which may affect the lungs and usually spreads quickly as an epidemic. The pros and cons of routine injection against influenza are complex. Managers should develop a policy which should be worked out in consultation with GPs and the local public health department. This policy should be written down and agreed with residents.

Anaemia

A resident who is anaemic lacks the normal supply of haemoglobin in the blood which leads to a shortage of oxygen throughout the body. He or she may look pale, lack energy and may suffer from palpitations, breathlessness, swollen ankles and sometimes a poor memory. Anaemia may also be a sign of other conditions such as kidney disease or cancer, and so a proper diagnosis needs to be made.

In some cases, once anaemia is diagnosed, it may be important to maintain regular treatment, and residents may need a gentle reminder to keep taking their tablets.

Varicose veins

Mild varicose veins can usually be managed by light Class I support stockings. More serious cases may be dealt with by surgery, but usually there is a long waiting list, and a resident may have to have therapy in the Home with a gentle exercise programme combined with rest and Class II or III support stockings. Long standing varicose veins can cause fragile and discoloured skin around the ankle which needs careful watching because any slight damage to that area may lead to venous leg ulcers, as described on page 71.

Skin care

The skin becomes thinner as we become older, and conditions which are tolerable in youth or middle age may cause considerable distress to an older person. You should ask for medical advice if a resident's skin shows changes in colour, becomes bruised, irritated or broken. Treatment may also not be as effective – for instance, in eczema where cortisone creams may continue to get rid of the rash but may cause abrasions or allow infections to spread. When a person enters the Home, his or her skin conditions should be noted as part of their care plan. Anyone with diabetes is especially susceptible to problems with the healing of skin lesions, particularly on the feet. If a diabetic person develops a sore, an ulcer or a black patch on a foot, his or her doctor should be called.

Some elderly people develop a sensitivity to certain foods and also to medicines and skin dressings. If there is any change to a resident's skin condition, such as the development of a rash, you should inform the doctor as part of the monitoring process.

An itching skin is also not just irritating but may be dangerous because scratching the itch can cause bruising and ulcers. Sometimes the itch occurs without apparent cause and can be due simply to dry skin. Itches can also be caused by scabies, a skin mite which is hard to discover but can cause endless discomfort among staff and residents until diagnosed and treated.

Wounds and ulcers

There has been considerable research over the last decade into the diagnosis and management of skin disorders, particularly pressure sores and leg ulcers. While proper medical diagnosis and careful nursing supervision are essential, the guidelines on treatment suggested below and on page 172 may be of interest to Managers, as they are aimed at encouraging sufferers or their carers to take more responsibility in assisting with the healing process.

Leg ulcers are very painful and often have an unpleasant discharge and smell. About 70 per cent are caused by inefficient pressure or valve disorders in the veins of the leg. A few are due to low pressure in the arteries.

Venous leg ulcers have the best healing success rate, and residents who have them can contribute immensely to the rate at which they heal by lying down at regular periods during the day. They should make sure that their legs are raised to a level higher than their heart with the support of pillows. In addition they should record on a simple chart the number of hours they have spent in the 'legs up' position. This record keeping will help them to feel they are participating in the healing process.

Other ways of management include gentle exercise and massage, not standing or sitting in the same position for too long, wearing proper lace-up shoes rather than slippers. Residents with ulcers may need reminding not to scratch the ulcer which may itch, and to take care not to knock their legs or to constrict the back of the calf against a chair.

Strokes

A stroke is a haemorrhage from a blockage in a blood vessel of the brain. A mild attack may cause temporary giddiness or confusion and weakness in a part of the body for a few days. The resident's doctor will usually advise rest.

A severe stroke has dramatic symptoms which may include a headache, vomiting, loss of speech and a sudden or gradual loss of consciousness. Medical help should be called at once. A resident who is unconscious should be left on the floor with a pillow under the head. Dentures should be taken out, as they may obstruct breathing.

Management

The two most common results of a stroke are weakness in the body, often on one side, and difficulties in speaking. Physiotherapy can help to improve movement and restore self-confidence, while speech therapy can help someone whose speech has been affected. Having a stroke can be very debilitating, and residents need cheerfulness and encouragement to give them the will to persevere in their recovery.

Parkinson's disease

This is a nervous disease which causes stiffness and slowness of the muscles and can lead to a shuffling walking movement and heavy tremor particularly of the hands. This is often accompanied by a 'pill rolling' movement between the fingers. The condition can be alleviated, though not cured, by medicines. Exercise and physiotherapy may also relieve symptoms, but the disease is progressive and sufferers will eventually need more and more help in their daily life.

Epilepsy

This is caused by an electric disturbance in the brain. Although the condition often affects people before the age of 30, it may occur for the first time in old age. A severe epileptic fit is very distressing, both for the person and for those who witness it. The sufferer may become unconscious, have convulsions, pass urine and foam at the mouth. A resident who has an epileptic fit should be kept warm and dangerous objects taken out of the way. Otherwise the person should be allowed to recover without interference. Usually the fit passes into sleep and the resident may wake up confused and with a headache. He or she should be treated gently at this stage.

Today epilepsy can usually be managed by medicines. Any resident who complains of violent headaches and flashing lights or who appears to have any form of fit should see a doctor as soon as possible for correct diagnosis and prompt treatment. Sometimes the first signs of epilepsy are unexplained bed-wetting or episodes of confusion.

Glandular disorders

One of the most common of these is diabetes, a disorder of the pancreas which may come on in youth or in later life. The symptoms include: an increase in weight, itching around the urethra, ulcers on the feet, cramps in the limbs and, sometimes, blurred vision.

Most people who have been diabetic since youth are on a strict regime with a special diet and insulin injections or tablets. The diet usually excludes certain foods, such as fatty red meat, preserved meat, full cream dairy products and sugar. A resident who develops diabetes in later life may well be able to manage the condition through diet, though sometimes they will also require insulin. It is important that a resident who has been diagnosed as diabetic is given the diet they require, as diabetics tend to be overweight. Other complications are eye problems and the fact that their skin is slow to heal, particularly on the feet. For this reason they need foot care from a qualified chiropodist.

In later life the thyroid gland can sometimes be overactive or underactive. If tablets are prescribed, it is important that they are taken properly and in the right dosage.

Cancer

Any organ or tissue can develop abnormal cell growths which are cancerous. It is important to take seriously and notify the doctor of any changes in the physical appearance or well-being of a resident. In some very old people, cancers are very mild and have been known to last for over 20 years without causing serious discomfort. There are a number of symptoms which may indicate cancer and which need medical assessment. Among these are :

- hoarseness or difficulty in swallowing;
- persistent pain in the stomach or abdomen;
- changes in bowel habits;
- blood in the stools or urine or as a discharge from the vagina;
- an unexplained swelling, ulcer or wart which does not heal.

Cancer may also cause weight loss and persistent fatigue. Many of these symptoms may have other causes, so correct diagnosis is important.

Many cancers can be treated and cured if they are caught early enough, and the outlook is improving with modern research. Treatment consists of surgery, radiotherapy or medicines (usually called chemotherapy), or a combination of any of these. Any treatment of cancer must be monitored carefully and any resident who is undergoing any therapy will need loving care and practical support during this time.

Stomach and intestines

Common conditions involving the stomach and intestines include hiatus hernia, stomach ulcers, diverticulitis and bowel cancer. All these need diagnosis and treatment as soon as possible.

Any resident who has persistent digestive symptoms, difficulty in swallowing, stomach pains or alterations in bowel habits for more than two weeks should have medical attention. A resident who passes blood in stools should be seen immediately by their doctor.

Constipation is another common problem in later life, as the muscle in the bowel wall becomes less efficient. It may be aggravated by lack of fibre in the diet, overuse of laxatives, general frailty and sometimes social or psychological conditions – for example, not feeling able to use the toilet in private. The condition can range from a mild feeling of discomfort to impacted faeces, which call for measures to remove the blockage.

Any person with constipation should have a medical check to make sure there is no medical cause such as a blockage and for advice on how to deal with it. As a general rule, you should look to preventive measures. The first of these is through adequate fibre in the diet from wholemeal bread, fruit and vegetables, adding bran if necessary. In some cases it seems as if regular exercise helps in improving bowel movement.

In some severe cases of constipation the GP may suggest the use of a bulking agent which is taken with water and builds and softens the faeces. However, some older people find the grains difficult to swallow. In more severe cases suppositories or an enema may be necessary. Laxatives should always be used with caution.

NOTE   Both bowel and bladder problems may cause embarrassment and distress to a person suffering from them. Staff should not refer to these conditions in public, and should at all times treat the resident with sensitivity.

CORNWALL COLLEGE
LRC

Incontinence

Research suggests that while this may only affect 10 to 15 per cent of the general elderly population, it is common in residential homes. Urinary and bowel incontinence may be completely cured in some cases. In others, the person may be helped through training the bladder, better toilet facilities and the provision of suitable aids. In all cases, managers and care staff should work out the best way to manage incontinence through a well-thought-out programme, including daily routines tailored to the needs of individual residents, and giving guidance for staff on night duty.

Assessment

Any resident with incontinence of the bowel or bladder should have their condition assessed regularly. This is often a team approach, with care staff, the person's doctor and a continence adviser working together. To help diagnosis, you will need to compile with the resident a history and record of their continence/incontinence and general health. The medical or nursing team will then be in a position to check for physical or psychological causes and to draw up a plan of cure or management which may include exercises, diet, a routine for going to the toilet and the provision of continence aids.

Management

The physical environment of a Home can affect whether a person remains continent. Privacy is important, so are enough toilets which are accessible, clean and pleasant to visit, with good lighting and heating. Residents should feel able to ask a member of staff to help them go to the toilet without being made to feel a nuisance. If they have problems in getting to the toilet, they should have access to urinals or commodes – in all cases with their dignity respected.

There is considerable advice and support available for residents with incontinence. Some health authorities have appointed a continence adviser, who is a trained nurse specialising in the treatment of this condition. District nurses have also developed specialist skills. They or the local community health centre will advise you how to contact the continence adviser. There is also a Continence Advisory Service at the Disabled Living Foundation (see page 166 for address). Many organisations, including Age Concern, run short courses on managing incontinence, and there are also videos and self-study materials available.

People in residential care should be entitled to the same financial help with incontinence equipment as is available to people who live in their own homes. Some health authorities will supply equipment to residents in local authority homes but not to private ones. You should always check whether NHS supplies are available by asking the district nurse or continence adviser or the local community health council. In some areas of the country, however, the NHS provision is limited, and the best supplies have to be bought privately.

You should try to spread the cost by building into your annual budget a specific sum for correct clothing and bedding for continence management. You may decide that you will charge residents for incontinence supplies, and this should be made clear in your contract with them. It is also possible in some areas of the country to borrow equipment, such as a commode or raised toilet seat, from the local Red Cross, WRVS, St John Ambulance or the social services department. Some local Age Concern groups also have equipment to lend.

For a detailed discussion on how to manage incontinence in a residential setting, see *In Control* (details on page 175).

Care of the mouth

Good oral hygiene is essential for comfort and for helping the digestive process. Most older people have dentures, which should be checked regularly by a dentist to make sure they have not become badly fitting. Dentures should be cleaned daily, and residents with dentures should be encouraged to rinse their mouth to prevent infection of the gums or interior of the mouth.

Residents who are on Income Support are entitled to free dental treatment under the NHS, and those on low incomes may also get help with the costs, as outlined in detail in the book *Your Rights* (for ordering, see page 175).

Care of the feet

It is often hard for an older person to reach down and cut their toenails and look after their feet. Corns and bunions may make walking even more painful for someone who already has an arthritic hip or a bad back. Regular chiropody will help to keep residents on their feet. Care assistants can be trained to help residents with daily foot care, but they should be aware that they need guidance from a chiropodist for people who are diabetic. For more information about chiropodists, see page 97.

The *Foot Care Book*, also published by Age Concern England, has detailed information on foot conditions (see page 175 for how to order).

MENTAL CONDITIONS

One of the most common mental conditions to be found among older people is confusion and it is essential to find out what may be causing it. Any resident who becomes confused over a day or two should see a doctor urgently before their condition deteriorates.

Although the symptoms may appear similar, there are three very different reasons for confusion which are: depression, delirium and dementia.

Depression

Many older people suffer from depression, and it is extremely common in someone who comes into a Home leaving behind a lifetime of independence. Depression may also be caused by poor health, loneliness, grief at the loss of a partner, thoughts of impending death, chronic pain or just not being able to come to terms with general weakness and disability, which usually involves dependence on another person. Around 15 per cent of the elderly population as a whole may suffer from depressive symptoms, but this figure rises when people become more frail and dependent. Of these, between 3 to 10 per cent of people in a residential home are likely to suffer from a major depressive illness which can be helped by medical treatment.

Diagnosis

One of the key issues is to identify depression. It often goes undiagnosed and untreated because it is not always easy to distinguish its symptoms, which may be different from those of depression in younger people.

Some older depressed people cry a lot, they do not appear to enjoy their food – usually a major event in most Homes – and often complain of physical symptoms such as headaches and constipation, when the real cause is deeper. Depression may be misdiagnosed as dementia, since the person may be withdrawn, apathetic and confused. Other older people with depression may be querulous, awkward, irritating and stubborn, be very suspicious or even appear to suffer from paranoia. Another sign of depression is when the person avoids eye contact.

It can be very helpful in diagnosing depression to find out from relatives, friends or professional workers what the 'normal' behaviour of the resident used to be and if there has been a marked change in behaviour. While there are many atypical ways depression can show itself, early identification will help effective treatment. The more you are able to help the doctor in his or her diagnosis, the better the chances of recovery.

Management

This should always be part of an overall care plan. It may include drug therapy or electroconvulsive treatment (ECT), and individual counselling and group therapy are also used. Loving care and attention from care staff will help raise the person's self-esteem and help them feel that they are not alone and that their problems are understood. Where possible the aim should also be to improve a resident's physical health and give them control over their own lives.

Delirium

This is due to an organic disease and common causes are chest or a urinary infection, heart disease or a stroke. Some medicines may also cause delirium as a side effect. When the cause of the condition is diagnosed and treated, the confusion will pass.

Dementia

This is a disease of the brain which causes progressive loss of memory and also affects a person's personality and behaviour. Often moving into a Home appears to precipitate dementia in a new resident which they may have been able to mask in familiar surroundings. Other signs of dementia are disorientation and the resident being muddled about where he or she is. The person may lose judgement skills about things like crossing the road and may start to wander and forget how to find the way back to the Home. Wakefulness at night is also a sign of dementia. Perhaps the most disturbing symptoms are aggressive behaviour, childishness and anti-social behaviour (masturbating in public, nose picking, etc).

Equally frustrating for staff members to deal with are the person's repeated questions about daily regimes such as mealtimes. Managers should ensure that staff members have adequate training in understanding the distressing behaviour of dementia sufferers and that they have an opportunity to discuss their attitudes towards severely confused residents.

Dementia affects one person out of ten over the age of 65 and one person in five over 80, so in a residential home the proportion of people suffering from Alzheimer's type dementia or multi-infarct dementia is likely to be high. Any resident whose memory is getting worse or who develops signs of confusion should be seen at once by their GP for assessment – a sufferer whose condition is not recognised is likely to deteriorate.

Management

While there are various therapies geared to helping someone with confusion or dementia, general management is carried out in the daily life of the Home. One residential home owner, where most of the residents suffer from Alzheimer's disease, makes sure there is always time to talk to someone who may be distressed.

Owner 'Sometimes one of our residents is frustrated or angry – they may say they want to go home to see their mother. If you try to stop them going out they just get more angry, so we never confront the resident and tell them they can't go. I find the best way is really to talk to the person in a gentle and kindly way, perhaps I just walk along and chat and try to regain their confidence. I may try to re-orientate them or even distract their attention. Usually the person calms down and stops trying to get out of the Home.'

In cases such as the one described above by the Home owner, the person may have feelings of distress but not know what has caused them because of a short memory span. The feelings then become attached to a similar event, perhaps from childhood which makes the resident want to go to their mother for comfort.

You can often pick up clues as to what a person with dementia is trying to say by listening carefully when they start to speak, and by observing the emotions that go with it, such as anger or frustration. For example, if you ask a question of someone whose memory span is only 30 seconds, they will remember the question for the first few words and then forget it. But their emotional response will continue, and you may therefore still be able to work out what they were trying to say. This can also happen in any kind of communication. Further suggestions about relating to residents with dementia are covered in Appendix 2 on page 171.

Consultant 'In my ward recently I asked one of my patients how she was, and she looked distressed and said. "All but the staring, the eyes!" I thought perhaps she was having some sort of hallucination. Then I looked round the ward and saw that everyone was looking at her and realised she was quite upset by being stared at.'

More formal ways of helping someone with confusion or dementia are through Reality Orientation Therapy (ROT), Validation Therapy and various group activities which may include reminiscence and music therapy. These need skilled handling. The community psychiatric nurse will be able to give you advice on the most appropriate therapy for residents in your Home, and there are a number of useful books on the subject (see 'Recommended Reading').

Reality Orientation Therapy

This is a method of bringing the person back to the present, to their current 'reality'. Care staff, members of the family, etc repeatedly give the person cues about the environment, and remind them of the date, the time of day, what they are wearing and so on. This approach is useful for people who have mild or moderate confusion.

However, ROT is not always appropriate and may be both stressful and harmful if carried out inappropriately. When a resident is upset by being brought back to reality, ROT should not be continued. Someone with dementia may be in such physical or psychological pain in their current present that they do not want to remain in it – they prefer to retreat to happier days.

Validation Therapy

As brain damage progresses, some older people may not be able to relate to ROT at all. With such residents, the most promising recent treatment is Validation Therapy. This means trying to understand what is behind the person's confused talk. For instance a statement such as 'Fred (my dead husband) has been here all afternoon' may really mean 'I've been thinking about Fred all afternoon and he feels very close.'

Research psychologist 'As speech becomes worse, language becomes more symbolic, almost poetic and must be understood in a new way. Universal themes of 'parents', 'children', 'home', 'work', 'loving' and 'being loved' are still understood in severe stages of dementia. Severely demented persons will often surprise you in that they will speak about these themes even if they say very little else. They draw on a lifetime of experience and not just the short-term memory.'

To be effective, staff should understand the principles, and Validation Therapy should only be carried out by people who are properly trained in its practice. This may be carried out in groups or individually.

Sufferers in different stages of dementia should not be grouped together.

Research has shown that people within each stage are able to communicate with each other, but may become very distressed when put with someone whom they recognise as worse than they are.

KEY POINTS

- Keep a look-out for signs of depression among residents, especially those who are new to a Home.
- As soon as you suspect depression, obtain medical advice and ensure that prescribed treatment is carried out.
- There are different causes of confusion, and these should be established as soon as possible. Some kinds of confusion can be cured.
- Mental stress and some medicines can cause memory loss and confusion which is not disease related.
- Although dementia cannot yet be treated, good management can improve a person's quality of life.
- A community psychiatric nurse or district nurse can give professional support with all mental conditions.

THE USE OF MEDICINES

All the medicines in the Home prescribed for individual residents are their property. They should never be administered to anyone else. The Home should provide all residents who are capable of looking after their own medication with a lockable cupboard where they can store their medicines along with their valuable possessions.

If a member of the primary health care team advises you that a resident is not capable of looking after their medicines, you may store and administer them. Keep all medicines in their original dispenser, with the name clearly marked.

Care staff should never mix prescribed medicines with those from a previous prescription, or with medicines belonging to other residents, even if they appear to be the same. This is the way errors occur. Similar medicines may have come from different batches, the contents may have been altered, or they may be of different strengths or have different expiry dates.

Medicines for residents unable to look after their medication should be locked away and given in the amount and frequency that the doctor prescribes.

After the death of a resident, or if they leave the Home, you should destroy or hand back all medication on the advice of the doctor.

The book *Know Your Medicines* has complete details about medicines used by older people. This is also published by Age Concern England (see p 175).

KEY POINTS

- Medicines are the property of the resident for whom they are prescribed.
- All medicines should be kept in a locked cupboard and only be handled by the resident or authorised care staff.
- Medicines should never be mixed with similar prescriptions.

COMPLEMENTARY THERAPIES

There are many other ways to maintain or improve health in later life, some by so-called 'complementary' therapies, which often have a psychological value. Some are being tried in the general care of older people. If a resident requests complementary treatment, you should suggest that they write to the Institute of Complementary Medicine (address on page 166) for information about a local practitioner, stating which therapy is required and enclosing an sae.

Managing pain

Many older people suffer pain in some measure from a wide variety of causes. Chronic pain usually has its ups and downs and is sometimes hard to alleviate. Depression may make it worse. If someone suffers from acute or unexplained pain, he or she should be examined and the cause dealt with promptly if possible.

People vary greatly in the amount of pain they can endure. Tolerance is high in an emergency, sport, battle and when being rescued. Tolerance is low if one feels lonely, without friends, depressed or helpless. Many older people

84

feel like this much of the time. People also often stoically endure pains that could be alleviated, if not banished. There are of course a number of pain-killing drugs which may be useful if given correctly.

Some alternative methods of managing pain are suggested below, where the person is encouraged to develop from being a pain victim to being a pain manager. Research has found that sympathy between therapist and sufferer can have an important effect on the relief of pain.

Acupuncture

This may be used only by qualified practitioners for a number of conditions, mainly pain relief. Some doctors also use it as part of the medical care they give. While acupuncture may not be suitable for the very frail, it can give effective relief to some when correctly administered.

Joint mobilisation

This includes heat treatment, mechanical vibrators, electrical stimuli, hydrotherapy and exercise. Different types of therapist may be involved, including physiotherapists, osteopaths and trained masseurs. Chiropractic involving strong manipulation and thrust of the joints is not appropriate for someone who is frail.

Altering the state of mind

Here, the person is encouraged to take their attention away from the pain. This can be done in several ways, including special relaxation techniques which focus attention on different parts of the body, starting with the feet and moving through the legs, to the trunk and upper body. Meditation, listening to music or any activity where the attention is directed away from the self may have a similar affect. Part of pain management is also not fighting it, to stay with the pain but look beyond it in a positive manner through changing attitudes. This may also help to close the pain 'gate', so that less pain is actually transmitted by the neurological systems.

Massage

Although some people do not like to be touched, it is surprising how many people respond to hands on their shoulders, placed in an unthreatening way.

Daughter in law 'One time we visited my mother-in-law and gave her a kiss and a cuddle when we said hello, and she said, "you know, apart from when you come to see me, the only other person who touches me is the lady taking our exercise class." And she said, "that's sad, isn't it?"'

Massage soothes tension, helps muscles to unknot and brings a sense of well-being. Animals raise their heads for a stroke though not many people in a wheelchair risk doing the same. But humans do respond to touch, indeed it is often a way to communicate with someone who is confused, unhappy or ill. A gentle massage, perhaps just of the back of the neck or the arms or hands, can bring a great sense of communication and bonding.

District nurse 'When I give something even as simple as a massage on someone's hands, I 'centre' myself, just concentrate on the other person. And by doing so, I am giving them quality time. I'm not rushing around and doing other things. It helps my stress levels too. I have often trained care staff and even families to do basic massage. There's no need to strip off. If you are not sure of someone's reaction, start with your hands on their shoulder, and then move to their arms or hands if they seem happy with that.'

Aromatherapy

If massage is combined with aromatherapy, that is, massage with essential oils, it also adds the sense of smell and can bring back memories and feelings from the past. This is very suitable for older people because it is gentle and yet effective. It works through smell and touch, which are still strong in old age when sight and hearing may have grown weaker.

District Nurse 'Smell is evocative and nostalgic and it will take people back to times they like to remember. You may be able to experiment and find a particular smell that brings back happy memories and use it to scent their room. Essential oils can give a special ambience, particularly when incorporated with touch – perhaps in a gentle massage.'

Sometimes this nurse uses her essential oils to change the atmosphere if, for example, she has to dress a leg ulcer which is not healing. It takes the person's mind off the ulcer, which is often painful and smells bad, and gives time for talking about other things. Aromatherapy is well worth trying out in a Home and is something care staff can do without extensive training.

Some therapists also add to the atmosphere created by the scent of essential oils by putting on a tape of natural sounds such as birdsong or running water. This can have a very soothing and comforting effect.

KEY POINTS

- Medicines relieve pain best when doctor and patient work closely together and communicate well. Try to encourage this.

- Alternative therapies are being used to supplement conventional medicine.

- Smell and touch are two senses many people respond to and can enjoy into old age.

- There are more important sides to running a Home than keeping to the timetable. Always encourage staff to make time for residents.

- Many alternative therapies have a beneficial effect on the well being of a resident and may help in pain relief.

- Advice about the use of massage and essential oils can be obtained from the primary health care team.

Managing a Home

This chapter is aimed at managers and owners of Homes which are up and running. You may already know that good management is a balance between a number of factors which sometimes conflict and that your job is to find that balance and maintain it. While you will hopefully have experienced the rewards of running a successful business, as a manager you are accountable in ways that demand skills and expert knowledge in several areas:

- the principles of care
- good business practice
- liaison with social and health care teams
- the development of a management style
- the ability to communicate with, lead and motivate staff

Marketing is another essential aspect of successful management. It is a skill which most small business proprietors are not trained in. For more advice on marketing, see the chapter 'Starting Out'. As marketing is something that you have to do constantly, you should go through the checklist on page 22 at regular intervals when you are planning your strategy for the following year.

GOOD BUSINESS PRACTICE

A residential home is a substantial investment. A private home will have equity of anything from half a million pounds to over a million. Much of this money will have been borrowed from banks, corporations and private individuals. If the Home belongs to the owner outright, there is still the need to ensure that there is proper accountability.

When Homes are registered or inspected, the inspectorate often ask for properly audited accounts by independent auditors. So every manager/owner will need to be thoroughly familiar with all aspects of running a business, and will experience many of the same problems as someone offering residential accommodation in a hotel or guest house.

There are a number of publications and organisations which offer advice to businesses of all sizes. There are also Government and other agencies which you can approach for personal consultation (see list on page 165). But you will get the best out of professional advice when you understand the basic principles on the financial side, what you are liable to pay out and receive when you are running a business.

Controlling the money

When you first set up in business, it is most likely that you drew up a business plan and a cash flow forecast like the one on page 170. Have you kept one and brought it up to date? You should be using it already as part of financial control. If your business does not have a detailed plan, it is advisable to draw up one.

Sources of income

These obviously will vary according to the type of Home and the amount of outside financing a manager can expect. Managers of local authority homes will have a budget allocation as part of the local authority's community care plan. The income for Homes in the voluntary sector may come from several sources including fees from individual residents, Income Support, grants from the relevant charity and contracts with the local authority. There may be supplementary income from other services provided within the community.

Private owners will also rely on contracts with the local authority to provide a certain number of beds in addition to generating their own sources of income mainly from residents' fees and Income Support.

For details about the funding of care after April 1993, see 'Introduction', page 13.

Outgoings

As with income, outgoings will vary according to the type of Home. To avoid the problem of underestimating the amount of working capital needed to keep your Home running, you can use the following list of outgoing expenses as a model:

Salaries and wages for staff

Tax and national insurance

Proprietor's or partners' earnings

Insurance premiums

Subsistence

Linen and household expenses

Medical and nursing aids

Repairs and maintenance

Capital equipment

Running costs – electricity, gas, telephone, etc

Transport

Special events

Membership of professional associations

Subscriptions to care journals

Contingency funds

To help you plan ahead and maintain financial control, you may find useful the short explanations outlined below of some of the more complicated outgoings. As with all aspects of financial control, you should of course get expert advice.

Taxation of owners/proprietors

The method of paying tax for a sole proprietor or a partnership is different from that for a private limited company, so it is worth taking informed advice. A sole proprietor or partnership pays tax under Schedule D, which is paid retrospectively, two years after the end of the financial year. A private limited company pays corporation tax yearly, and the directors are taxed under PAYE, which means that tax is deducted from their salaries every month as it is for employees. The taxes payable and national insurance payments may be significantly different depending on which business set-up is chosen.

Staff salaries and tax

When employing staff you have a statutory obligation to deduct tax and national insurance from your employees' wages. This has to be paid over to the Inland Revenue, each month, together with the employer's portion of national insurance, for each employee. In order to do this, it will be necessary to register with the Inland Revenue which will supply you with the necessary tax, national insurance, sick pay and maternity pay tables, together with a payslip booklet, etc.

As there are various legal aspects involved in paying salaries (eg statutory sick pay and maternity pay) you should get professional help.

If you are concerned about having to pay VAT, you should note that Homes registered under the Registered Homes Act 1984 need not register for VAT and are exempt from charging VAT on services which they provide for their residents.

Occupational and private pensions

This is a another complex subject which requires expert advice. You may decide to set up a company pension scheme, even though you are not obliged to do so, and you may also want to consider a personal scheme for yourself and for staff members. There is general information about occupational and private pensions in the Age Concern publication *Your Taxes and Savings* (details on page 176).

Plan ahead

The annual budget should set out clearly what you foresee will happen over the next twelve months, month by month, as shown in the cash flow forecast on page 170. Cash is the life blood of a business. Your cash flow forecast should include a detailed breakdown of all estimated income and expenditure for the forthcoming year in the areas listed under Outgoings, plus any others which are relevant.

The major errors or problems to do with cash flow forecasts are:
- overestimating the amount of income to be generated;
- underestimating the time of receipt of residents' fees;

- underestimating the amount of working capital required to keep the business running;
- not reviewing and revising the forecast throughout the year;
- avoiding talking to the bank manager when early signs of cash difficulties are foreseen.

To prevent these errors from happening, you need to keep accurate financial management information, so that you will know what happened in the past year at each stage in your plan. Checking your current position regularly against the budget or target set will help you to control the business. For instance, if you have overspent in one area and underspent in another, you will need to examine all the budgets carefully and re-allocate resources. Check up on care as well as financial targets.

By having the property regularly revalued by a surveyor, you will be forewarned about any unexpected item of depreciation which could throw a business into the red. You may need repairs to the roof, new furniture, better health care facilities or redecoration, which are required by the registration officer before renewing your registration.

Your annual cash flow forecast should have a contingency sum to allow for unexpected costs. Check that this is enough and when you draw it up, make sure that you allow for any building or interior work to be done during the coming year. You can control your credit balance by keeping a check on all outgoing invoices. Unpaid invoices that remain unnoticed can have a very unhappy effect on a cash flow forecast.

Avoiding difficulties

If you have been over budget in several areas, you will need to look again at your business strategy as a matter of urgency and discuss it with your bank manager. At this stage it is also very helpful to bring in an independent adviser or trouble shooter. You may then have to consider various options, such as:

Raising residents' fees.

Utilising staff resources in a different way.

Diversifying and offering some services to the community.

Changing your facilities to attract a different clientele.

You will need to think through each option carefully, noting not just the financial implications but what effect it may have for yourself, the staff, the care offered and the well-being of residents. For example, you may decide to raise fees, only to find that some of your residents could not afford them and that they are now above the maximum sum payable as set by the DSS, so that you would, in fact, lose revenue instead of gaining it. For details about funding after April 1993, see 'Introduction', page 13.

KEY POINTS

- Good practice means good financial planning and keeping control.
- A cash flow forecast agreed with the bank will provide a sound basis.
- You will need to keep forecasts up to date.
- Compare targets and forecasts regularly with what has taken place.
- Always think through all the financial implications of any changes you plan to make in the running of the Home.

WORKING WITH LOCAL SERVICES

As a Home manager, you already keep in contact with a number of people and authorities. It is worth making a serious effort to get to know all these different people, and to be willing to ask and take advice. This will help your business as well as provide for better care. The people with whom you will come into most contact outside the Home are from the social services (including the inspection unit), the primary health care team and other support services as well as voluntary groups or other interested individuals.

Here are some guidelines to help you use local services effectively:

- compile a list of local services provided by statutory and voluntary bodies so that you have somewhere to ring in an emergency;
- make personal contact with the people involved in providing these services;
- welcome visitors to the Home and get to know them personally – invite someone in for a cup of coffee;
- follow this up with a list of names of GPs, district nurses, social workers, physiotherapists, etc, who come to the Home regularly.

Help with training

Outside bodies have a number of functions. On the care side one of the most important is in training staff in special types of care – more important than ever as those living in residential homes become more frail.

Training sessions given by a member of the primary health care team are sometimes part of regular in-house training, but also occur as the need arises, for instance, when a resident requires special care. Someone with pressure sores has to be turned over in bed several times a day. Pressure area care needs sensitive handling, turning and positioning. The district nurse can explain how this should be done and should monitor the care assistant on his or her visits to make sure it is being done correctly.

Another common need for training is in continence management. The district nurse or sometimes a continence advisor, who is also a trained nurse, sets up a regime for taking a resident to the toilet and checking on the amounts of fluids passed at different times of the day. She or he will also provide charts for the care assistant to fill in.

Not every Home has in the past welcomed the addition of such time consuming work for their care staff, but it benefits the manager as well as the residents.

District nurse 'My view is that it is in the interest of the manager to follow our advice, because they will get a good reputation for the quality of care that Home gives. If they choose to ignore professional advice, then the quality of care deteriorates and word gets round.'

Social services departments

The organisation and structure of social services departments varies considerably from one local authority to another. Generally these departments have some responsibility to provide practical and psychological support to people in the community by reason, for example, of frailty, poverty, abuse, illness and physical or mental disability. They are increasingly developing structures that enable their staff to work in specialist teams. This is in response to the community care legislation and to that concerning children with disabilities.

Social workers

As a result of the social services restructuring in some areas of the country, managers of Homes (both private and voluntary ones) will liaise with social workers operating in 'adult' teams whose work is likely to be with older people. Frequently social workers play an important role in helping these people to decide which living arrangement is best for their future. Social workers are, therefore, likely to be key professionals involved in admitting residents to your Home. You will need to be able to work closely with them and to eventually take over the 'case' once a resident has settled in.

Occupational and physiotherapists

Occupational therapists (OTs) have a number of functions, which are aimed at improving the quality of life in a given environment. They are concerned with training people to acquire new skills or develop existing ones. Much of their work in a residential home is about helping older people with disabilities to remain active or become more able to do things for themselves and so get more out of life. An occupational therapist has a wide knowledge of aids and adaptations which can be made to Homes. Many OTs are also involved in organising group or individual activities in a number of ways.

Physiotherapists (Physios) are trained to treat disorders of muscles and joints with a variety of techniques, including massage, manipulation and heat treatment. Gentle physiotherapy can be of great benefit to older people. Physiotherapists work from a hospital or in the community from a health centre and should provide domiciliary visits if requested by a GP. There are also many who have set up in private practice for those residents who can afford private treatment.

Physiotherapists will also give advice on the most suitable aids for mobility, such as walking frames and wheelchairs. The district health authority is responsible for providing wheelchairs under the NHS, so if one resident has a particular need, try to organise a visit to a disabled living centre where the resident can try out and choose the most suitable chair.

Availability

Health and local authorities provide varying levels of domiciliary physiotherapy and occupational therapy services. Some authorities will view private residential homes as a legitimate use of these scarce NHS and social service resources. Others will feel unable to help. Contact your health authority's district physiotherapist or the social services senior occupational therapist to discuss your needs. If they cannot be met, you may want to consider employing a private physio or occupational therapist.

Primary health care team

This is the name given to all those who are concerned with the health and social welfare of members of the public in the community. The team may include as appropriate: GP, district/community nurse, community psychiatric nurse. The team is concerned with maintaining and improving the health of people in the community, providing emergency care, health education, screening for referral care, identifying needs of patients or clients and offering preventative measures. The primary health care team has an important training role, which includes care staff as well as students in their own disciplines.

All residents in a Home should have by law the same access to health services as people living in their own homes. This means they are able to use a doctor of their own choice and that you, as manager, should consult first with a resident's GP as the gate keeper of day-to-day health needs. There may be instances when you can call in a district nurse on a resident's behalf without referral to the GP if this is appropriate, ie if a resident's condition requires nursing rather than medical care.

The residents' right to choose their own GP does have some drawbacks – in one Home for instance, 17 doctors visit 68 residents! As a district nurse may also be attached to a GP's surgery, you may find 17 district nurses assessing and treating all those patients.

General practitioner

GPs of the residents' choice provide treatment, information about matters of health and referral to other medical and nursing services. Some doctors are part of a medical practice, but many are now part of a health clinic which offers several services. GPs prescribe medication for residents in their care and this is usually administered in the Home. (Injections, however, must be given by a district nurse.) Most GPs will visit residents in the Home, and it is helpful if you are able to supply details of any complaint by the patient, or symptoms which you or the staff have noticed. This is where good record-keeping proves its worth, because doctors rely on the information they are given to help them in diagnosis.

District/community nurse

These nurses are based at a health clinic set up by the local health authority or at a GP's practice. Each unit is managed by an experienced nursing sister.

District nurse 'I used to go to one Home to give insulin to three patients with diabetes. Gradually I found the manager was coming to me with all sorts of other problems, like incontinence.'

In such cases it makes more sense for the system to be rationalised. District nurses seem hopeful that in the future there will be one identified nurse per Home who will be the prime assessor to link up with the appropriate GP. This will mean they can build up an overall consistency of care. As residents become more frail, it will help their changing care needs to be assessed.

Some geriatric hospital departments have a community nurse who works as liaison between the hospital and the patient and assesses how fit and independent someone has to be in order to cope at home after being discharged from hospital. If this is the case, a district nurse may be requested to visit a resident to assist in the post-discharge period if there are nursing needs.

Most of the district nurses' work is in the community itself. As part of their nursing duties, they liaise with social services to ensure that the total needs of the individual are being met and there is no duplication or overlap in the provision of services to an older person. There are three aspects of their job which may involve a residential home: assessment of nursing needs, giving nursing care to individual patients and training care staff to carry out special care under their supervision.

Assessment

The district nurse, together with other members of the primary health care team, may be asked to participate in multi-disciplinary meetings, where it is decided what is the best care for their patients or clients, which may include a recommendation for residential care. This is usually the admission practice in local authority homes and some voluntary homes. It does not always apply to private homes. The district nurse can be a valuable source of advice once a person has been placed in a Home, by assessing nursing needs and making referrals to services like physiotherapy or occupational therapy where appropriate.

Community psychiatric nurse

Community psychiatric nurses (CPNs) may be available and are based either at psychogeriatric hospital units, health centres or elsewhere. They work closely with the consultants in hospital and can be a valuable source of ongoing support and advice to managers of Homes where there are residents who suffer from mental health problems which result in behavioural difficulties in the Home.

Chiropodist

Even though NHS chiropody should be available to older residents in Homes, it is very scarce, and the reality is usually to look for private treatment. You should enquire about private practitioners' training. If they are State registered, they will use the letters 'SRCh' after their name.

As NHS chiropodists are in short supply, it is not usually possible to get their help with routine foot care such as toe-nail cutting. In some areas, a nailcutting service may be supplied by a footcare assistant, recommended by a chiropodist. Your local Age Concern group should also know whether this service is available.

Dentist

Residents are entitled to the same dental services as other members of the community. They should be encouraged to visit their dentist for regular check-ups even if they wear dentures, as these can become badly fitting.

The community dental service may operate a home care system for residents who are housebound. Their GP can make a referral for this, or the Family Health Service Authority will have information about the service.

Speech therapist

To get NHS treatment, the resident's GP will need to make a referral. As the availability of NHS speech therapists is very patchy, you may need to contact a private therapist. The organisation Communilink has nationwide information about appropriately qualified private speech therapists (address on page 166).

```
KEY POINTS
```

■ Get to know the services available to support you within the community, and make personal contacts where you can.

■ Make use of the skills of practitioners and therapists who visit the Home. They can be a valuable source of advice and training for care staff.

YOUR MANAGEMENT STYLE

Not all businesses are run the same way. They vary according to the personality of the owner or manager, the size of the business or organisation, the nature of the business and, of course, its personnel. The two most common methods of organising personnel are within a strict hierarchy or where people work in teams within a matrix or network.

A good manager is able to bring together both these approaches. Clearly he or she will be the only person with the knowledge to take certain decisions because they may have business or financial implications. But improving communication with your staff and making their jobs more satisfying can only be of benefit to everyone concerned in a residential home.

Working in a hierarchy

This is the traditional method of running an organisation. Everyone has their place and their rank. If you have worked in the civil service or the medical or nursing professions, you will have encountered a strict hierarchy. The advantages are that staff know just what they have to do, and aspects of the work can be planned and organised. The disadvantages are that this kind of work may not be fulfilling for those on the lower levels. Staff often feel, and are, out of touch with senior managers, they are not invited to contribute their ideas, and imagination and creativity are often stifled.

Working as a matrix

This is a more modern approach which new industries such as the media, high tech or communications often employ. There are of course line managers, but the emphasis is on the task force and teamwork. It means that quick decisions can be made because people in different areas have similar levels of responsibility and do not have to refer upwards for every decision. If your background has been in the social services, you are more likely to have worked in this way. The disadvantages of a matrix are that high level decisions may not be made because managers are not given enough information, or the organisation may become so informal that important work is left undone. On the positive side, it gives staff the chance to contribute their ideas and skills, develop their potential and feel a worthwhile part of their own business.

Communications skills

As a manager, you may find it helpful to take a course in communication and negotiation skills, which are run by a number of organisations as well as colleges of further education. There are also several good books on the subject. You may learn something new for yourself and it should prove invaluable in training your staff. Courses cover topics such as:

- listening skills and body language;
- being assertive or saying what you mean without being aggressive;
- finding out relevant facts about a subject;
- taking notes and writing reports;
- making a presentation to a meeting;
- making out a case for negotiation;
- understanding the aims of the other person;
- preparing counter arguments.

As local authorities implement a policy of contracting out care to the independent sector, private home managers will be made accountable for the services they provide. The better your own communication skills, the better you will be able to present a good case to licensing, registration and other authorities. Good communication skills are also essential in your contacts with staff and the residents in your care.

Time management

This is covered more fully in the next chapter as part of good office administration (see page 115).

Self-motivation

This is linked with setting goals and targets. Regular checking of your current practice, financial and care targets are usually strong spurs to keeping yourself motivated. However, you also need to feel supported by those who work for your or with whom you come into contact. Regular meetings and discussions in the Home as well as meeting your peers and other professionals will help to provide support.

KEY POINTS

- When organising staff, you may feel more comfortable working in a hierarchy.
- The matrix approach to organisation puts the emphasis on teamwork.
- Communication skills are a useful tool for dealing with all outside bodies and people.
- Check that you manage your time properly, including time for yourself.

BUILDING A TEAM

Building a good team is one of the most important tasks of management. It provides the manager with back-up, it uses the skills and experience of staff in a way which is fulfilling, and it provides a framework in which the Home can function effectively. But who is in your team? You, the senior staff, the care and catering staff. Is there anyone else?

Manager 'The key element is that ultimately there is one team, and that team includes the residents. It's one big heaving mass – all the parts are interconnected. There is nothing going on in a Home that isn't going to have an impact on something else in terms of people's relationships.'

This goes back to the model of a matrix organisation, a network of people where you, as manager, are in touch with all the connecting threads. A team is more than a group of individuals who happen to work together with rules laid down by their manager. There are a number of predisposing factors, such as the leadership of the team. This is often decided by situation, not simply by position or protocol, ie the longest serving member of staff is not necessarily the best team leader. The team should also recognise that it is part of a wider organisation, which in this case includes the residents, with whom it is important to develop relationships.

All teams take on their own identity, and have the power to impose their own standards of behaviour and performance, even if these are against the wishes of management. A successful leader understands this and takes the team's needs into account. The leader should involve the members of the team in decision making, communicate efficiently with them as a group and as individuals, brief them regularly and consult them before taking decisions which affect them.

If you take over the management of a Home, it is quite likely that you may inherit members of staff who have been working in the Home for a number of years and who have their own ideas of what should be done and how to do it. It can be very frustrating for a new manager.

Manager 'When I took over, some of the older members of staff were stuck very much in the task orientated side of care – and I have some sympathy for them because they've seen so many changes. They would rather see a client sitting passively in a chair in clean clothes than somebody who is quite happy with a bit of egg down the front of them and doesn't want to be disturbed.

'Well, when I saw this attitude I redesigned the work programme – I looked at what each person did and I wrote out my new methods and had a meeting and explained it to everybody. They were all very suspicious and very, very reluctantly decided to have a go. To them it was an implied criticism of the way they had been working. And of course my scheme fell flat on its face, not so much because staff were trying to undermine it, but because they were genuinely confused. It lasted all of about two weeks! In my view, you have to get people to talk about it, make their own suggestions and then you can begin to make changes.'

There are several ways of getting people to talk about team work, through informal chats with individuals, through meetings which you do not attend, and through regular formal meetings. This will give both sides a chance to discuss any problems they are facing, their training needs, etc.

Make use of meetings

The purpose of holding a meeting is to exchange information, to consult, to give a chance for people in a junior position to air their views, to get ideas to improve the running of the Home and to get volunteers to participate in activities, outings, etc.

Some staff meetings are formal affairs, with a set agenda, minutes and formal recommendations. Other managers prefer a less formal approach, perhaps asking their staff in for a cup of coffee at 10.30 am when the residents are having theirs. This different approach to meetings is part of their management style and can apply in large as well as smaller Homes.

Some Homes have very few staff meetings. They tell staff what to do individually or through their supervisors, who also hold few meetings. However, most managers find meetings helpful in anticipating problems that may arise. They can find out what their staff are thinking and feeling, and meetings give staff the opportunity to be involved in the Home and share ideas.

A specially called meeting should have a purpose, otherwise it is a waste of time and can cause frustration and become devalued. Most meetings are concerned with:

- giving information;
- gathering information;
- persuading people;
- solving problems;
- taking decisions.

Meetings need a leader or facilitator if they are not to get out of hand or lose their value. Usually this is a manager or a deputy. The leader has to have a clear idea of the purpose, to plan it, which means bringing or circulating any relevant information, papers, etc. Conducting the meeting effectively without doing all the talking is also the leader's responsibility, as are keeping it to time and making sure that everyone has a chance to contribute. Everyone involved should know what the meeting is for, and the leader must ensure that it does not get sidetracked from important issues.

Manager 'In my view, the Home is a working environment for staff and they have just as legitimate a contribution about the colour of the lounge or the colour of the loo paper as the residents.

'Meetings can centre round the practical things – has Mrs Patel taken her medication today, what time shall we hold the fire drill next week, all that sort of stuff. But that may not leave time for considering why you may be doing this or to question the assumption that Mrs Patel should have this particular kind of medication, or be helped with a walking stick instead of a frame, or whatever. I think the most successful Homes are those where all things are questioned all the time and staff feel free to contribute to the discussion.'

Have an agenda

This may seem rather a formal way of going about a regular monthly meeting, but it does help managers and staff to think beforehand about points for discussion – it stops the meeting going off at a tangent. The agenda serves to remind all those attending of the topics to be discussed, and why, and it also serves as the structure for the discussion.

During the meeting

Make sure everyone contributes, especially the silent ones, whom you may have to draw out. Be specific on the questions you ask. If you are considering installing a lift, for example, ask just how many residents actually would use it, as distinct from those who could. Staff would then be able to consult residents before the meeting.

If you have called a meeting for a particular purpose, it is helpful to summarise what the meeting is for at the beginning and what you hope to get out of it. This may include an item on which people have strong views, and often it can be hard to separate fact from opinion. In such cases, the following approach may be useful:

Seek information and ask people to keep to the point.

Summarise the situation without giving your opinions.

Diagnose any problems based on the facts provided.

Seek opinions and evaluate them – including your own.

Summarise what has been agreed and what action should be taken.

Make sure this is understood.

Stress the positive aspects of the conclusions reached.

Problem areas

There are always people in meetings who are aggressive, talk too much, say very little, think they know it all and so on. You need to find a way of using their contributions.

A most useful booklet published by the Industrial Society on effective meetings describes a range of personalities, from the bulldog, who always wants to win and needs to be isolated, the horse or monkey who have contributions to make but need to be restrained, to the fox, who likes to slip a banana skin under everyone's feet, including yours as leader. The advice is, don't tackle foxes directly. Ask the group what they feel about their contributions. Group wisdom can often serve as a useful ally!

KEY POINTS

- A team leader should involve members of the team in decision making.
- Staff must have an opportunity to suggest changes themselves in the way the Home is to be run.
- Meetings give staff members a chance to share ideas and be involved in the Home.

LEADERSHIP SKILLS

There are a number of ways in which you can develop your own leadership skills, which start from having a clear idea of your aims and objectives. Leadership means being able to stand aside from your daily work and look at the ingredients which do not always work well or run smoothly. Weak leadership can lead to inefficient use of resources, waste of time, poor communications, low morale and ultimately loss of business. While it can be hard to analyse those areas in which you lack skills as a manager, it is essential to do so in order for your business to develop and prosper.

Looking at it from a positive angle, the main areas of good management are considered in more detail below:

- taking decisions
- delegating tasks

- supervising staff
- dealing with staff grievances
- responding to residents' complaints

Taking decisions

Much of a manager's time has to do with making decisions – or putting them off. All too often we put off making a decision because it may involve us in conflict, we do not have all the relevant facts or we just don't have the time. Decision making can usually be broken down into five questions:

- What is the problem?
- What information do I need to make an informed decision?
- What are the possible decisions I could take?
- What are the consequences of each decision?
- Which course of action fits into my overall strategy to provide the best care within the constraints of budget, staffing, etc?

If you find it hard to decide between two or three different solutions, take time to think through their consequences in detail. Build up a picture in your mind of where decision 'a' would take you in a year's time. Do the same with solutions 'b' and 'c'.

The next stage is to consult. Talk over your possible solutions with people who will be affected by them. Take professional advice. It often also helps to talk over your decision, if it is a major one, with an outsider. Which solution convinces them, and is that the one you feel most comfortable with?

Once you have taken a decision, explain to those concerned what decision you have reached, and why. Finally, check again that the decision will actually work.

Delegating to others

This is an area which managers who have been used to working in a hierarchy often find difficult. They don't like to give up power, perhaps because they think someone else may not do it as well, but often because they enjoy power. This may be good for a manager's ego, but not always for their bank balance. If you find it hard to delegate, ask yourself some honest questions as to why.

- Are there tasks that someone else could perfectly well do?
- Can you think of a member of staff who could do them?
- If not, could they be done after training?
- Are there things which you know need doing but you never seem to get around to?
- Have you left enough time for your own pursuits?
- Are there members of staff who need stretching and who would benefit from taking on more responsibility?
- Are there residents who would like to be stretched and could take on some responsibility?

If you have answered 'Yes' to most of these questions, it is likely that you bear most of the responsibilities of the Home, and you should think seriously about delegating some of them.

A close look at how you run the Home may help you feel more confident to delegate some of the managerial tasks, which include: having clear and attainable objectives; being a good supervisor; and motivating staff.

Clear and attainable objectives

These include the objectives of the Home, objectives for care, and goals to improve that care. Tell your staff your reasons for doing certain things, and give them a chance to discuss your ideas.

Good supervision

Supervisors, whether their title is senior care assistant or assistant manager, are usually responsible for specific areas of work. In some Homes, the manager/owner will carry out some of these responsibilities, which include:

- understanding the aims of the Home and the principles of care;
- leading a team;
- induction of new staff;
- Health and Safety regulations.

A supervisor is often the link between care staff and management. At one level, they may stand in for the manager when dealing with social workers, the Inspectorate, families of residents and so on. On the other level they may assist or stand in for care staff helping a resident with a walking frame. A supervisor needs a calm manner, to be mature in his or her approach to the job, and to work closely with and motivate the team.

Supervisors need to be aware of what jobs need doing, and to be flexible enough to see where a care assistant is genuinely doing something for the good of a resident and when they are avoiding essential work. As the supervisor goes around the Home, he or she will be considering the following points:

- What are the work priorities for this shift?
- What points must I check on during each working period?
- Which care assistants will need special help, training or supervision?
- Will staff on the next shift have all necessary information?
- What training do I need to give or arrange for staff?
- Do I need training to improve my supervisory skills?

Residents' complaints

In a Home where emotions may be very near the surface, you may sometimes have to deal with complaints which arise from poor communication or basic misunderstandings and which can be sorted out once you know all the facts. Sometimes there is no clear-cut solution.

Regulations 9 and 17 of the Registered Homes Act, 1984 set out guidance on the duties of managers with regard to complaints. When a resident makes a complaint, they should be given information in writing on the steps being taken to investigate it, and also the name and address of the registration authority. They may also take the complaint further, if they wish, to the registration authority or, if it is a local authority home, to the Ombudsman. These people will certainly want to know how the complaint was investigated and what action, if any, has been taken.

When you receive a complaint from a resident, a member of their family or an outside visitor, there are certain steps which should be taken. Listen to the complaint, show concern and write down the main points. Ask questions to establish the circumstances of dissatisfaction. If possible ask the resident to suggest a solution, but do not commit yourself to it at this stage.

First, investigate the facts, such as the time when an incident occurred and whether there were any witnesses, etc. Check whether policy or regulations have been broken and whether something like this has happened before. If so, how was it resolved? If you believe there is a genuine case for action, decide whether you can handle it or, if you are not the manager, whether you should involve the manager.

Decide what you are going to do about the complaint and how you might deal with the complainant's reaction. Write down how you will put your decision across and if you are in any doubt, take advice.

When you communicate your decision to the individual or their representative, ensure that you have privacy and that there will be no interruptions. If the decision is not acceptable, you should discuss what further action can be taken, or the procedure for an appeal.

Later on, you should check that what was agreed should happen has actually taken place and that the resident feels that his or her complaint has now been settled.

In dealing with complaints, both managers and staff should remember that this is part of quality control – residents must be encouraged to talk to anyone in the Home about things they do not like. After all, they are paying for their care. If managers or staff feel threatened by complaints, they should ask for training so they understand the necessary procedures to follow.

Staff grievances

The initial procedures for dealing with staff grievances should be similar to those for residents – all grievances should be taken seriously even though they may appear to be trivial or unfounded.

It is useful to know the areas where staff may have problems in their work and to give them a chance to talk about them. Often a situation can be defused before it reaches the stage where a formal procedure is the only solution. The areas will vary according to the individual Homes, but may include:

- residents with special problems;
- unfair treatment by another member of staff;
- a personality clash between a member of staff and a resident.

Grievances may also occur if managers make changes in the daily routine or conditions of employment without previous discussion and agreement – for instance, changing shift times, asking people to do overtime at short notice, and so on. This is where an understanding of the personalities of your staff is very helpful. Some are willing to be flexible, others like to know exactly what is expected of them and are thrown when a situation suddenly changes.

It is of course never possible to foresee all potential sources of grievance, and it is important to have a strategy to deal with them and to ensure that all members of staff are aware of the correct grievance procedures.

Managers in the public sector and in many larger Homes in the voluntary sector have a procedure laid down which applies to employees in that organisation. A typical local authority grievance procedure contains a number of sensible steps designed to settle a grievance as quickly as possible (excluding those which relate to pay, disciplinary action, pension schemes, national insurance contributions, etc).

- The member of staff raises the grievance with their supervisor, with a union official present if they desire this.
- The supervisor replies verbally to the member of staff as soon as possible, and in any case within seven days.
- If the employee is dissatisfied, he or she may take it up with a representative of the union to raise with the supervisor.
- If the employee is still not satisfied, the employee or his or her representative submits the grievance in writing to the manager/chief officer, who has to reply in writing within seven days.
- If the matter is not resolved, a meeting of all interested parties is arranged with a local authority personnel officer.
- A final appeal may be made to an appropriate committee of the local council or authority.

An employee using this grievance procedure is given access to all records and correspondence in their file which relate to the grievance.

Procedure for smaller Homes

Most small Homes, ie those with less than ten members of staff, have no formal procedures for dealing with staff grievances, and these are handled by the manager or proprietor. While the procedure given above may not be appropriate for the small Home, the principles may be adapted.

The employee raises the matter with the supervisor, who should reply verbally within seven days. If the employee is not satisfied with the decision, they should approach the manager directly and should at this stage have the opportunity to ask for a representative. This could be a union official if they are a member, or someone who may be able to put over their point of view.

A manager who is unable to resolve the grievance at this stage may consider asking for advice from a professional association or the local authority inspection office, which will have a wider experience of dealing with staff grievances. The employee may make a final appeal to a consultative board if one exists, or the manager may decide to bring in an outside arbitrator.

Talking and listening

In developing their leadership skills, managers should of course be very aware of how they speak to residents and staff members and whether they give enough attention to listening to people. These are part of the communication skills outlined on page 99, but they also require extra attention and sensitivity.

For example, whether you are delegating certain management responsibilities to a staff member or discussing the day's menu with a resident, you should remember to speak at a speed which the other person can understand and use simple words. This is particularly important when communicating with someone from an ethnic minority group. You should also remind staff to take care about speaking clearly to residents and to each other. Tone of voice is another important aspect, especially when talking to a partially sighted resident or someone with dementia. You can put across sympathy, anger or firmness by your tone of voice.

Being a good listener involves a lot of different things. You not only hear the sounds the other person makes when speaking, but you must also listen for hidden meanings. For instance, does a care assistant's complaint about her rota perhaps relate more to her dissatisfaction with her poor social life?

When listening to residents, remember that many of them were brought up feeling it was wrong to show their feelings. When a resident complains that someone else's visitors always make such a lot of noise, that person could really be saying that he or she wants to take a nap or that they are feeling left out and would welcome something to do.

Managers who are good leaders are just as aware of sensitive communication as they are of the more business-like aspects of good management.

KEY POINTS

- Decision making can be broken down into questions to ask yourself.

- Good management involves giving responsibility to staff members who would benefit from this.

- Many managers benefit from training in good supervision.

- Be aware of your attitude about residents' rights to complain about aspects of the Home.

- Grievances from staff members should also be listened to with care.

- Pay attention to the words you use and your tone of voice when communicating with staff members and residents.

- Being a good listener can add greatly to effective management.

The Daily Running of a Home

All businesses benefit from having an office that runs smoothly and which provides managers with essential back-up through a qualified administrator, efficient systems and suitable technology. In running a residential home, supporting your staff is of equal importance so that they feel confident about their tasks. This is particularly important in our multi-racial society where you may have both residents and staff members from minority groups in your Home who may be confronted by racist attitudes.

In this chapter we discuss all these topics and also outline the skills required in giving care to sick residents or to someone who is dying. The practicalities of good hygiene practice and providing a nutritious diet for residents are also covered.

Some of the guidelines given in this chapter are the result of recent thinking on good care practices, and relate to the management skills discussed in 'Spotlight on the Residents' and 'Managing a Home'

GOOD ADMINISTRATION

The efficiency of a well run Home is centred in the office and the systems you apply. In 'Setting up a Home' we stressed the importance of good administrative systems and practice. Some of these may be required by the inspection unit, others will help your business practice.

A secretary/administrator

Research has shown that a part-time high calibre secretary will provide much more support to a manager than a full-time typist. Secretaries are trained to process information, use word processors and information technology, have good communication skills, do the book-keeping, payroll, etc, and carry out much of the routine work that a manager may not have time to do – or indeed have the skills.

Good secretaries can do a lot more than just look after the paperwork. They use their skills to arrange meetings, take minutes and type them up, look after your diary, liaise with residents' families and the community health and social services. Of course a manager can do all these things, but they take up time. The more you can delegate routine work, the more time you have for the essential management tasks outlined in this chapter.

People returning to work after bringing up a family are often a good choice for work in a residential home. They are mature, have administrative skills a younger person may not have, and are likely to be good at dealing with people. Someone in this age group may also find that working in a Home suits her because hours can be flexible and a part-time job may be all that is needed. You should make sure that anyone you appoint has the necessary skills to operate new technology, even if you do not operate any at the moment.

A filing system

Every office has paperwork which cannot be computerised, so you need a good system, which you and your staff can understand and work. Confidential files, such as residents' financial affairs and staff records, should be kept separately.

You will also find it helpful to have a 'bring forward' system, which helps you keep tabs on all the different things to be done like care assessments, details of training programmes, fire drills, etc.

Office technology

This can transform the work of a small business and usually includes a word processor or personal computer, fax, telephone and answerphone. If your Home is a large one, you may also need a bleeper or a mobile telephone, so that you can leave the office and also be reached in an emergency.

With the proper software packages, you and your office staff can enter up and store information, run the accounts and do your financial planning. A cash flow forecast is simple to update when it is set up on a spreadsheet on your computer. If one item has to be altered, the adjustments will be made automatically to the bottom line of the spreadsheet at the touch of a button.

Manager 'In my last office we did all the work by hand and it took ages. But my advisers said get a computer, and a year later I invested in one – it was the best thing since sliced bread! I took a course to find out how to work it, and my accountant advised me on setting up the accounts. I seem to use it for just about everything – all the residents' records, bits of paper coming in about this new Act. My diary is there and I have a spreadsheet for future planning.'

Record keeping

As in any business, it is essential to keep up-to-date records. As a model for these records you can obtain pre-printed forms for schedules, rotas, etc from Tower Printers at the address on page 167. With the new inspection procedure, the registration office could well ask for a great deal of information about records which could be held on computer. These might include:

A daily record about each resident.

Case records for every resident.

Details of residents' money and valuables to be stored.

Staff handover book regarding resident care.

Records of all medicines kept in the Home.

Menus, diet sheets, records of meals served.

A record of fire drills and equipment testing.

Staff records (references, contracts, pay levels, etc).

A record of accidents involving staff and residents.

NOTE   Under the Data Protection Act, residents have a right to see any information you hold about them on computer. As a matter of good practice, the same should apply to written records.

Schedules

Good schedules will help you plan ahead, and make sure that staff are available for all duties. You will need to have:

Work rotas organised on a monthly basis.

A yearly calendar of engagements and events.

A weekly chart showing regular commitments.

Schedules of regular meetings with all staff.

If your schedules are computerised, it will not cause much extra office work to change them and issue new schedules.

The manager's time

It is useful when allocating staff duties to also estimate your own use of time. It helps if you have clear priorities in your daily work which are written down, not just held in your head. Writing down your routines can also prove invaluable to your staff if you are away or ill, and someone else needs to take over for a while. Things will continue to run smoothly if your priorities are set out clearly, so that your assistants are aware of them.

One important priority is to set aside some time regularly for office work. This is often hard for managers, especially when they are also owners. Use your time in the office for thinking, planning and checking. As mentioned earlier, your efficiency will benefit from employing a competent office administrator or secretary for routine work.

Try to make one or two daily 'rounds' in the Home, to monitor staff and make sure residents get the care they need. Don't make these rituals – they should appear to be spontaneous, rather than an 'inspection'. You should also hold regular meetings with staff, and try to ensure that these are not cancelled through pressure of work. Another very important aspect of time management is making time for recreation, both privately and with the residents, as a participant not a leader. Managers should also take a break from the Home and go out for pleasure, not for shopping or home visits.

Staff rotas

A residential home has to provide staffing cover 24 hours of the day, 365 days of the year. This is a lot of hours to fill. Most Homes have two shifts during the day and one at night. In drawing up staff rotas, you need to take into account peak times of work which correspond with the residents' requirements (see the chart on page 40) as well as those of individual staff members.

Rotas may vary, depending on where the Home is situated and on the availability and safety of public transport. Very early or very late travel may be, or feel, dangerous, especially for female staff. Staff need to be able to rely on their hours of work, and changing rotas are unsettling for them as well as the residents. Homes which plan their rotas well in advance provide continuity and save valuable time and resources. You need to consider the following points carefully when drawing up rotas:

– Consult staff if you propose to make changes to shift patterns.

– Regular time off will help staff plan their private lives.

– Plan rotas particularly carefully for staff members with school age children.

– Have sufficient temporary staff available, including senior staff, for emergencies or holiday periods.

– Do you have provision for a 'skeleton' staff?

– Be sure to build in time for meetings and training.

Decide on the shift pattern to suit your Home, which will include the times of each shift, number of hours worked, and how many core staff you will need on duty. When the shift system is in place, you will need to review it with your senior staff and at meetings to make sure it is working smoothly.

A key worker system

Many Homes give one care assistant special responsibility for the care of a small number of residents, usually between three and five. A key worker system is not usually practical where the number of residents is small, but you should certainly consider introducing it, perhaps for a trial period, if there are sixteen or more people in your Home. Your registration and inspection office or a trade association, if you are a member, should be able to suggest a Home in your area with a well-run key worker system, so that you can talk to the manager, see how it works for yourself and discuss the pitfalls and advantages.

Usually a key worker is involved with the new resident right from the start. They may visit the resident in their own home and they help them settle in the residential home. The key worker will assist in drawing up a resident's care plan, take them to special clinics or hospital visits if possible, and generally act as their advocate if necessary.

Key workers build up a special relationship with their clients, they know their likes and dislikes, the types of TV and radio programmes they enjoy, when they prefer to get up, how they like their hair done, who their relatives are, and so on. This is likely to add to job satisfaction as well as improving the efficiency and quality of care.

In care, as in all walks of life, occasionally there is a personality clash. Under these circumstances there is no point in persuading the member of staff or the resident that they 'have' to get on together. It is much simpler and more satisfactory for all parties concerned to avoid a confrontation. Arrange for the member of staff in question to concentrate on working with other residents, and encourage the resident to take up an activity which will take him or her out of the immediate vicinity of the member of staff. Usually a bit of distance between two people smooths over any difficulties after a while.

KEY POINTS

- Keep routines flexible, so that residents do not feel pushed around.
- Office efficiency is an essential part of good management.
- Good office organisation will give you more time for the jobs that only you can do.
- Write down your priorities rather than carrying them around in your head.
- Shift rotas known in advance will provide the most stable care.
- A key worker system gives residents the feeling that they are of special importance to someone who understands them.
- The key worker also has the chance to build up a special relationship with residents.

SUPPORTING YOUR STAFF

Giving support to staff during their daily work is essential – this means both emotional and practical support and training, so that they are confident in what they do.

Emotional support

As you will be aware, caring for older people can bring anger, frustration, heartbreak or boredom, as well as enjoyment, friendship and the rewards of knowing you are helping someone. Everyone, managers and care staff alike, will experience some of these feelings during their work. As a manager you need to be aware of all these different feelings and give your staff support in expressing or coming to terms with them. There are many ways you can do this, as outlined below.

Mentoring

Arrange for an experienced member of staff to take a new one under his or her wing for a few weeks to help not just with practical tasks but also with the emotional stresses and strains. This is in addition to an induction programme.

Meetings

Bring your own feelings up at meetings if it is appropriate, and encourage staff to talk about theirs. If there is a problem, discuss possible courses of action. New staff in particular should be encouraged to give their opinions. This will also give you an opportunity to evaluate their contribution to the Home.

The open door

Many managers encourage their staff to feel free to drop in and talk to them at any time. If the offer is there, it may not be taken up, but it helps staff to know that you are there for them.

Use expert advice

If one member of staff is having particular difficulty, arrange for them to talk to someone from outside the Home who may have professional counselling skills. Use them yourself too – managers are likely to need a confidant just as much as their staff do.

Practical support

The senior member of staff on duty will provide the main support for care assistants during their day-to-day tasks. District nurses, occupational therapists, etc are also trained to give practical advice on anything from lifting techniques to suggestions for an afternoon's recreation.

Training

Staff also need proper training before they start work and once they have started. There are several ways you should provide this – through an induction course which you are legally obliged to give staff, through day-release courses at a local college, through outside training agencies and through in-service skills training – which may also lead to National Vocational Qualifications.

Many Homes hold regular weekly and monthly training sessions in all aspects of running the Home, from taking responsibility for a fire drill to managing incontinence. This provides an opportunity for experienced as well as new members of staff to learn new skills, or hear about a new way of doing routine work.

Training is covered in detail on pages 155–163.

Combating racism

We live in a multi-racial society, and we all need to be aware of the conscious and unconscious attitudes or prejudices which can affect our behaviour. Racism is best met in an up-front way by discussion and action, rather than by reaction to prejudice after it has occurred. If your Home is in an area with an ethnic mix, or if there are some residents or staff from a minority culture in your Home, you may need to look at your own attitudes and set up good practices. There are a number of ways in which this can be done, but it is not always easy.

Check out your feelings

Do you give out racist attitudes? How much time do you spend with people from ethnic minority groups to get to know them? Have you considered the unique contribution that staff members from an ethnic group could make to the Home? Do you encourage such people to apply for jobs and give them responsibilities equal to those of their white colleagues? Before appointment, do you consider what training may be made available to assist someone from a minority culture to meet the job requirements? After appointment, do you give them the support they may need?

Talk about racism

Set the topic of racism as a lead item at a staff meeting, so that members can air their fears and discuss the effects that racism has had on them. Be prepared to listen to both sides – each perhaps feeling threatened. If members of staff from ethnic minorities would like it, also meet separately with them to check that they are not subjected to racist practice from other members of staff or from residents.

Find role models

One of the best ways of combating racial prejudice is through example. Make good use of black and ethnic minority professionals, trainers, and key staff in the training programmes that you arrange in the Home.

Make sure that all staff receive training in 'combating racism'. Often the use of a white trainer will serve as a good role model here.

Keep the residents informed

You may find it necessary to talk to residents as well as staff when a care assistant from an ethnic minority is coming to join the Home. You may not be able to change older people's attitudes, but you can make it clear that the expression of racism is not acceptable.

Residents as victims

Make sure residents from ethnic minorities are not subjected to racism. This can be achieved in two ways: through example – by the way you treat each person with dignity, and by making sure that all staff know that racist behaviour is not acceptable in your Home.

Homes should also have appropriate written reference material about minority groups' practices in regard to diet, religious festivals, etc. Telephone numbers for further information from organisations such as the Jewish Board of Deputies can also be useful.

KEY POINTS

- Staff members need support in their work from a variety of sources.
- Practical advice from the primary health care team can be invaluable.
- Training will provide a framework for staff to develop their skills and confidence.

- Examine and express your own commitment to anti-racism.
- Many racist attitudes are caused by ignorance and fear. Give people the opportunity to express these openly.
- Arrange training to combat racism.
- Enable both staff and residents to respect their major religious festivals and their cultural and dietary needs.

ADMINISTERING CARE

Most managers are used to preparing routines and working to schedules. The skills in managing good care come in between the schedules. The following section will focus on hygiene, diet and giving special care.

Daily tasks

There are daily routines which have to be carried out in the Home each day by the staff on duty. The tasks included are:

- serving meals and clearing them away;
- bedmaking and collecting laundry;
- clothing and dressing;
- bathing;
- helping residents to go to the toilet.

From the residents' point of view, it is important that daily tasks are not carried out in a rigid or mechanistic fashion. Managers should remember that some residents may have special needs because of their religious beliefs or cultural background. Try to make it a general rule that all the systems are flexible.

Manager 'There are basic tasks such as assisting people out of bed, into bed, bathing, etc. But once the rush is over, which is from early morning till about ten o'clock, much of the time is spent talking to the residents or working with them, perhaps on their care plan. We have a key worker system here, so each care assistant spends individual time with a small number of residents.'

Voluntary worker 'In some Homes I visit, the care seems so mechanical. You have to wake up, have breakfast, sit in the lounge, have a morning cup of coffee and so on. In such a static routine it is quite difficult to see how people can function in an individual way. That was brought home to me very forcibly when two sisters had to go into a private residential home because one, who was used to looking after her very arthritic sister, got a very bad leg ulcer which prevented her from coping in their own house. I knew them well and was very aware of their personal habits – how they conducted their lives.

'When they entered the Home the three of us were involved in tussles with the manager because in that Home, once the residents were downstairs, they were not allowed back in their bedroom. The two sisters found that extremely restricting. They were only there for a short time so they moaned and put up with it. But for those people who are there all the time, their day is often dictated by what suits the staff.'

Good hygiene

Hygienic practice is important in any residential setting, and is particularly necessary in a Home for older people. They are more prone to infection and disease because their natural resistance is weak. Some of the most common conditions which older people suffer from are caused or aggravated by poor personal or domestic hygiene.

Residents' hair

Brushes and combs should be washed weekly. Ask staff to keep a look out for very dry scalp and for head lice and to treat these conditions if necessary. Encourage weekly hair washing. Looking good is important for self-respect, and a visit from the hairdresser provides not just a personal touch but a feeling of well-being.

NOTE   Some residents may wish to wear their hair in a special way for religious or cultural reasons.

Washing hands and face

Care staff's hands should be clean when preparing or serving food. It is essential that they wash their hands after visiting the toilet or helping a resident use the toilet. Ask them to check that residents also wash their hands.

Wash basins in the lavatory will help here, and this is something which Hindus and other Asian residents will require.

Staff should also take special care in observing good hygienic practice when handling any soiled or infected materials, as outlined below.

See that clean towels are freely available (and not restricted to once a week). Ask staff to encourage residents not to wash their faces in bath water.

Laundry arrangements

There are strict regulations governing these which include the provision of adequate bed and other linen, proper sorting, laundering and disposal arrangements for laundry and waste materials and a separate laundry area which is away from the kitchen area or any place where food is prepared or served. You will need a good washing machine, which can stand up to frequent use and high temperatures.

All linen should be changed and washed at regular intervals. Blankets should be able to withstand washing at high temperatures, and duvets should be washable and fire retardant. Residents should have access to a personal laundry service.

All staff should take great care in the handling of linen and soiled clothing to prevent the spread of infection. Soiled linen should be stored in disposal bags or colour-coded containers for separate washing, which must not be by hand.

Some managers contract out their laundry services. If you prefer this option, you should make sure that holiday periods are covered, and that the services meet the health inspectorate's regulations.

Waste disposal

It is important when sorting waste material to check that all sharp objects such as razor blades, needles or syringes have been put in protective containers.

The health regulations also lay down how waste or infected material should be stored and collected for disposal in colour coded bags:

Black bags, for normal household waste.

Yellow bags, for all waste for incineration.

Yellow bags with a black band, for waste which is preferably incinerated.

Light blue or transparent bags with a light blue inscription, for waste which should be put in a sterilising oven before disposal.

All containers used for holding soiled linen or waste should be washed, dried and disinfected thoroughly. Staff should observe personal hygiene and wear disposable gloves when handling infected linen or waste materials.

Kitchen hygiene

Cloths used in the kitchen should be kept and laundered separately from cloths used to clean toilets and bathrooms. Kitchen surfaces should of course be kept clean.

Guidelines for the proper storage and handling of food must be part of good practice in Homes, as discussed on page 28.

Clean air

A smell of urine is unpleasant and unnecessary. A stale smell often occurs when residents wash their tights or pants and put them on a radiator to dry. Soiled garments should be washed as soon as they are removed and dried in a laundry room. Soiled household linen should be removed before it dries out, and incontinence pads should also be disposed of immediately.

Using the toilet

Helping residents, or reminding them, to go to and from the toilet is a daily part of the care staff's duties. Discuss with them and with the resident a suitable day and night routine to help ensure dry clothing and bedding. The following checklist may be helpful:

- Make sure that two members of staff are available for helping a resident to the toilet if required.
- Check that the lavatory, including seat and pan, is clean and that there is enough toilet paper.
- After lifting someone from a chair or helping them on to the lavatory, allow for maximum privacy.
- If it has been requested, ask care staff to observe the contents of the lavatory pan. Report change of colour or blood in the resident's urine.

- Check that the resident's clothing is in place before they leave the lavatory.
- Care staff and residents should be sure to wash their hands.

NOTE   Men may not like being taken to the toilet by a woman, nor a woman by a man. Managers should be sensitive to these feelings.

Diet and nutrition

It hardly needs to be said that the type of food that is served and how it is cooked and presented will contribute greatly both to your residents' health and to their enjoyment of life.

Older people have somewhat different nutritional needs from those of the average adult population. On the whole they need the same nutrients but in a smaller quantity. Often when people come into a Home they have been used to poor eating habits and may have developed fixed preferences. Some may be following outmoded diets, have lost the will to care for themselves or have dental problems, which make it hard to chew. Factors such as malabsorption or disease may also substantially alter their nutritional requirements.

Older people may feel very resistant when faced with a change of diet, and, as always, a balance should be kept between respect for residents' wishes and what nutritionists consider best for older people. Discuss possible changes in diet and menus with everyone concerned. You may find it helpful to bring in a dietician for some training sessions on nutrition in old age.

Diet for older people

Proteins

These are needed for the growth, maintenance and repair of the body. They are present in fish, meat, dairy products, eggs, nuts and vegetables such as peas, beans and lentils.

Carbohydrates

Unrefined carbohydrates provide fibre to help prevent constipation and are a source of energy. They are present in wholemeal bread, wholegrain cereals such as porridge, jacket potatoes, bananas, etc. Refined carbohydrates such as white flour and sugar provide calories but no fibre.

Fats (animal and vegetable sources)

These are a concentrated source of energy which may be of particular use to a frail elderly person with a tiny appetite. However, fats should normally be eaten sparingly to prevent overweight.

Vitamins

These are present in most foods. Light cooking of vegetables preserves their nutritional value, especially vitamin C. The most common deficiencies in older people are Vitamins C and D. Some older people are prescribed a vitamin and mineral supplement, but as excessive vitamins can be harmful, this should only be included as part of a care plan on medical advice.

Minerals

These are essential to good health and include: iron, present in meat and eggs, which is needed by red blood cells to keep the blood healthy; calcium, contained in dairy products, which is important in preventing brittle bones. Some practitioners consider zinc useful in preventing behavioural and sleep disturbances, night blindness and immune deficiencies.

Fluids

These are very important for older people, who should drink at least 3 pints (1.5 litres) daily and more in hot weather. The more frail residents may need extra encouragement to keep up their intake of fluids.

Fibre

This comes entirely from plants and binds water and other nutrients together and produces bulk in stools. It aids elimination of waste products and so helps to prevent constipation. Fibre rich food is filling and cheap and includes beans and lentils, oat products, cabbage, broccoli, Brussels sprouts, parsnips, beetroot, citrus fruit, apples and bananas.

However, fibre may be harmful to people with certain diseases. Wheat bran in particular prevents the absorption of essential nutrients. Check with a dietician or doctor if you are unsure about a resident's diet.

Giving special care

There are occasions when the daily routine of care for residents has to change because they are sick or dying. The book *Taking Good Care*, also published by Age Concern England, has a comprehensive section on both these aspects of care. The following remarks are particularly applicable to managers.

Care of a sick person

The district nurse will be responsible for setting up a care routine for a sick resident. As mentioned earlier, they will train or supervise care assistants to undertake necessary routine tasks, such as washing, lifting, care of the mouth and teeth, dealing with pressure areas and any other type of care the patient needs, such as help with feeding. As manager, you should be ready to give care assistants support and back-up where necessary, and make sure that the district nurse is coming in regularly to check the patient's condition.

Care of the dying

Residential homes are considered as a home for life, and most residents normally stay there until they die, unless the level of care required cannot be catered for in the Home. Death is bound to disturb people's feelings and fears. It is important that care staff have training in dealing with it, both with regard to the best type of physical and emotional care to give dying people, and to help them cope with their own feelings and those of the other residents.

It should be stressed that even though a person is apparently unconscious, he or she may be able to hear what is being said. Everyone at the bedside or in the room of a person who is terminally ill should be very careful not to say anything that could cause them distress.

Talking about death

This is still one of the taboos in our society and there are no rules about what should be said or how death should be approached. As with many fears, talking about it does provide an outlet. When a doctor tells a patient that he or she is terminally ill, that person will need a great deal of support and love from care staff. In reacting to death, most people will go through several stages and may move back and forth between them. The stages include:

Denial that death has been mentioned.

Anger directed at God or a particular person.

Withdrawal, turning their face to the wall.

Acceptance of death while maintaining dignity and self-respect.

At each of these stages residents should be encouraged to express their feelings and talk about their fears. You or the staff may not be able to allay them, but if you listen and are available to give comfort, including holding their hand or stroking their forehead, you can show that you are with them in their distress.

Staff and residents may also need the opportunity to talk over and express their feelings about death. It is helpful if you arrange some special counselling for staff, and maybe yourself, to prepare them for what will for most be a distressing part of their work.

After someone dies

There are several procedures to carry out after a person has died. If the death is unexpected, you may need to inform the next of kin and call the person's GP. In some cases the doctor can sign the death certificate. If the doctor has not seen the patient within two weeks of death, the coroner may need to be notified, and a post-mortem will be necessary in some cases. The body must be laid out and prepared for burial, which may need to be done according to a specific religious rite; check with someone from the appropriate faith or ethnic group if you are unsure of what to do, as mistakes can cause great distress.

Relatives and residents may wish to pay their respects to the deceased person, so you should allow time and privacy for this. The resident should be treated with dignity in death, and it is suggested that the coffin is taken out through the front door of the Home – though you may wish to tell other residents in case they prefer not to witness this.

There is also a funeral to arrange, according to the late resident's religious faith or wishes. This task may fall to you, and you should be aware that the person who makes the arrangements with the funeral director may become responsible for the cost even if they are not related to the deceased person. Financial help with a funeral from the department of social security is only available where the dead person has left insufficient money to cover the cost. If you are advising the relatives of a resident who has died, they may be eligible for help with funeral costs if they are in receipt of income support, housing benefit or community charge benefit, and they should be aware that there are certain capital limits which relate to their savings.

For more information on arranging a funeral, see Age Concern England's Factsheet 27 available as explained on page 178. Relatives dealing with a dead resident's assets may find it useful to read Factsheet 14 *Probate – Dealing with Someone's Estate*.

KEY POINTS

- Daily tasks must be carried out by staff with sensitivity and flexibility.

- Good hygiene in Homes for older people is particularly important for the health of residents.

- Many residents need help from staff in getting to the toilet at routine intervals.

- You should respect residents' wishes when recommending a healthy diet.

- The district nurse will set up arrangements for special nursing care in the Home and should train and monitor care staff if necessary.

- People who are dying who appear to be unconscious can often understand what is being said around them. Make sure that staff know this and avoid causing further distress.

- Don't let death be a taboo subject. Older people and staff need to talk about it and discuss their fears.

The Quality of Care

When we talk about quality of life or quality goods, we usually have some sort of picture in our minds – a fantasy perhaps: sitting by a Mediterranean harbour in the evening sunlight, dancing till 5.00 am at a disco, winning the pools, having a lazy Sunday morning in bed, wearing the latest trainers. Everyone has their own fantasy, their own idea of what quality means for them.

What is quality of life for someone in a residential home? Good health, someone to talk to, a cat to stroke? Or the feeling of being loved, not being in the way? Or could it be having a room of your own with your possessions around, a glass of sherry at 6.00 pm, knowing that someone is going to help you out into the garden afterwards?

Quality of life for an older person has fewer extremes than for the rest of us. They will be lucky to get to the seaside in Britain, never mind the Mediterranean. They won't be able to show off their expensive trainers in the high street. For some, every morning is a lazy morning in bed.

This chapter looks at how Home managers can build at least some quality into the personal care and the lifestyle of their residents. It will expand on ideas mentioned in earlier chapters and also examine the ways to monitor and control that quality.

THE HOME ENVIRONMENT

First impressions are important, and a residential home is no exception. What does someone new coming into your Home feel about it? Are there fresh flowers in the hall, or a just a few drooping potted plants? Do you smell furniture polish or urine? What colour are the walls – dingy and non-descript or reflecting light? Creating a friendly atmosphere which looks as if someone has cared need not cost a lot of money, but it pays dividends in helping people feel good. Does your Home have:

■ fresh flowers once or twice a week

■ good lighting from lamps and ceiling lights

■ clean curtains

■ a variety of pictures and ornaments on the walls

■ bookcases, books and magazines

■ some nice-looking pieces of furniture

Creating a friendly atmosphere

One reason a person's home looks different from an institutional one is because there is an element of the unexpected in someone's house or flat. Things are not always where you think they should be – there is clutter around. Although you would not want serious clutter in a residential home, you can achieve a creative feeling by having more things about than are strictly necessary – a wall with several pictures, some belonging to residents, chairs placed in groups, not all facing the television. A cat or dog can also add to the feeling of being in someone's home.

To help achieve an informal atmosphere you could:

– Ask new residents if they have something special they would like to have in the Home. It will still remain their private property.

– Have a stand in the hall for walking sticks, etc, which people can borrow.

– Look out for mirrors, hall tables, etc, next time you are at a market stall.

– Ask residents' friends or family members to help with ideas or objects to make a homely atmosphere.

Put out the welcome mat

A Home also feels lived in when visitors are at once made to feel welcome. Staff, as well as you yourself, should be willing to talk to visitors, find out what they want and take them to their destination. No one likes to be left on

132

an uncomfortable hall chair for five minutes while a care assistant goes to
fetch a member of the senior staff.

Keep up family connections

Some residents have regular visitors, some have very few. Encourage
residents' families or friends to visit them – get to know their names, find
out a few personal details. Make a point of stopping for a quick chat about
someone's dad or aunt if you pass them in a corridor and encourage care
staff to do the same. Most residents miss their families and these visits are
very important to them. If family members feel looked after, they will get
pleasure as well as giving it, and the resident will also benefit.

In many areas volunteers often come and visit people in residential homes
who have no family or friends. Some churches or religious groups organise
visits as well, and for pet lovers there is even a 'Visiting Scheme' whereby a
nice friendly dog will be brought by its owner to talk to residents and be
petted by those who wish.

Within a caring environment, residents will be able to feel cared for in other
ways, in their body, their mind, and perhaps also in their spirits.

Lifting the spirits

There are all sorts of ways to encourage people to feel better. The most
important are: giving time, not rushing someone who is slow – and most
older people are – listening to residents' opinions and taking them seriously,
being physically gentle. These are covered in more detail elsewhere in this
book.

There are other areas as well. Some help to take people out of themselves in
just a small way – by doing some gentle exercise, choosing the right clothes
for an outing, being able to reminisce with other residents, having a library
of easy-to-read books around and so on. A few suggestions are given below,
but there are many more which will be appropriate.

Stepping out

Centre on Aging 'It's never too late to take strenuous exercise. A group of
frail, sedentary 90-year-olds suffering from ailments including arthritis,
heart disease and high blood pressure and who lived in a residential home or

a hospital started high intensity weight training three times a week. After eight weeks, these people were between three and four times stronger and more mobile.'

This press report from the Centre on Aging at Tufts University, Boston, Massachusetts, brings home an essential point about exercise. Stronger thigh and calf muscles means your legs are steadier and give better support. Marksmen and women use weight training to give them a steadier aim – stronger arms and hands can help you hold a cup of tea without dripping it all down your front. All residents should have the chance to take part in exercise, from simple movement to the occasional old time dancing, if they enjoy it.

Visiting services

Everyone likes to look good, to make the best of themselves. If a resident is not strong enough to go out, you should try to arrange for services to be brought into the Home.

Owner 'I arrange for a chiropodist to come in every six weeks, and a hairdresser once a week. Residents pay for those services, everything else is included. A volunteer comes every Monday and she does some of the ladies' nails, puts nail varnish on. She's a lovely person, very chatty.'

Singing

This is good for the heart and lungs as well as for residents' spirits. Many Homes welcome local choirs or groups of young people who come and perform for them. Cubs, Scouts and Guides often arrange regular visits, as do local schools. If your Home has a regular singing group, ask them to involve the residents throughout – reminding them of the words if necessary, so that there is less performance and more singing along.

Nursery teacher 'Every two weeks Pauline, the deputy head, and I visit the old people in Queens Crescent. Pauline takes her guitar and we also take toys, paints and jigsaws for the children to use. They play quite unselfconsciously among the residents. Then we all sing – nursery rhymes for the children, old-time favourites for the older people. We encourage the children to talk to them, and some are very good. At Christmas all the children were dressed up, and we did a nativity play, and the old people were clapping and crying. Actually I was very moved myself.'

Outings and events

Owner 'We take them over to Blenheim Palace, just for coffee, and then go into the garden centre, because it's only one step down. And they can walk round a little shop. September we all go down to the local fair in the high street.'

Most Homes arrange outings from time to time – anything from a visit to the theatre for a matinee to a day out to the country. They may be hard work to organise, but are usually fun for both staff and residents.

Administrator 'We have a summer coach trip, where we go out to a local place of interest, have lunch and see some sights. Then we usually organise a trip on the river. Our local shops here are very good, they do special evenings for disabled people and our staff take anyone who wants to come down to the shopping centre.'

Local outings which are popular include going down to the local pub or fish and chip shop. Events inside the Home can provide a regular source of stimulation – such as draughts, chess tournaments, quizzes, etc.

Administrator 'We offer a wide range of other things for residents to do. They have whist drives, they play bingo, they'll do crosswords together on a blackboard, they'll play carpet bowls – that always causes a lot of laughter. Once a week those who are able are given the chance to make their own lunch. Then the occupational therapist also encourages people to paint or make wall hangings and so on. Altogether I should think that of our 37 residents, between a dozen and twenty are involved regularly each day in these activities.'

If you are in a part of the country where there is popular entertainment or where people come in for a local festival, you may also find visiting groups which like to entertain in local residential homes. You may be able to contact them through local theatres or entertainment venues, or a theatrical agency advertising in the *Yellow Pages*.

Reminiscence groups

Getting people to talk about the past helps them to use their memories in a constructive way. A group of no more than five or six meet for an hour or so to talk about events of the past. Usually an occupational therapist or trained care assistant acts as the leader. He or she will aim to spark off discussion though audio or visual aids. These could be records, old photographs, newspaper cuttings, a TV programme set in the 40's or 50's.

Photographs from earlier times are often on sale in bookshops or art shops. These are not usually expensive, and may evoke all sorts of memories. Some are available for purchase in packs from the Winslow Press. Help the Aged also publishes a reminiscence newsletter (addresses on pages 166–169).

Your local library can often provide access to local history records as can local authority activities officers. They may be able to lend out material about your area before the planners take over – pictures of clothes, shops, traffic, etc. Any of these can be a trigger to the memory.

Leading this kind of group needs training, and not all care assistants are comfortable in doing it. Reminiscences can disturb and distress. While it may be good for the residents to express their feelings, some younger people may find it hard to handle.

Reading

Reading can be a great pleasure for someone whose eyesight can cope   it keeps the mind going, and it can take you into another world. Local authorities are able to provide a library for the Home of books, both large print and ordinary ones, which are charged for on a regular basis.

Owner 'A lot of our residents here bring their own books, and often we inherit them when they go, so we have built up quite a good library – crime, novels, current affairs – all sorts. Last autumn our advisory council ran a very successful bring and buy sale with some of the residents, and we used the proceeds to get some large type books. We are in the country here, and people like to keep in touch. I'm sometimes surprised at the books I see around – quite complex political analysis.'

Being sociable

Even a small Home can have some sort of little bar which is opened perhaps two or three times during the day. Even if a resident should not drink alcohol for medical reasons, there are low alcohol beers and wines which make a pleasant change from the usual soft drinks. Some places have a 'happy hour' when residents are encouraged to have a drink with other residents and their family or friends. Some Homes seem to have a round of parties.

Owner 'As you can imagine, we have birthdays nearly every month, in fact there are two this month, and we always have a party. I try and get their relatives to come too. We have a bottle of sherry and it's really good. And then there's a club around the corner where they have afternoon teas.'

Food as a focal point

This is a major part of everyday life – often meal times are the highlights of the day.

Resident 'Food is very important indeed. I look forward to my meals very much. We have a cook who really has imagination – we may have the same meat but it's served in all kinds of different ways. She knows I like my food and several times the cook has come up to me and said "Can you think of a new dish for supper tonight?" I gave her one dish which is now called after my name!'

In one Home, the manager makes sure that there is always something in the way of food or drink throughout the day to provide a focal point.

Manager 'Every two hours there's something. I purposely space it out like that, so that at least people will speak and be spoken to. From breakfast to lunch is a long time, and if someone is feeling depressed and withdrawn, it gets them out of their room and into the dining room and gives them a chance to sit down and chat.'

Respecting feelings

This is linked up with realising that people are individuals at any age. Some people need and like being helped, others prefer to do as much for themselves as they can in dressing or bathing – and that gives time for other things like chatting.

Resident 'Sometimes I need a little tactful help, that's really all it is. I'm best with someone who lets me be free to talk as slowly or as fast as I like, or as much as I like. When you're over 90 you can't do what you did when you were younger and you've got to adapt yourself. But it does take time – it doesn't come easily'.

Relating to others

People living or working within any organisation may develop a relation-ship with the men and women they work among or come into contact with. Most people are supported by relationships throughout their lives, but, sadly, most people in a residential home have lost their partner. Sometimes they find new friends and even lovers in the Home.

Manager 'Two of our residents have a relationship, by that I mean a sexual relationship. There are quite a few close relationships between some of the women – they talk to one another, they support one another.'

A different manager found that residents started getting to know others when the sitting areas were made smaller so that it became easier to com-municate with other residents.

Manager 'I've noticed that if there are a lot of people sitting in a room they'll just sit there and won't communicate, whereas up to four or five residents will talk quite freely – they don't feel inhibited or they don't feel they are interrupting someone else's television or radio programme. Television can be a dead weight in a Home. I feel it should be available in people's rooms, but perhaps only in one public lounge, so that there is space for individuals to meet.'

In most Homes where there is a key worker system, the care worker will relate to each of the residents as individuals, not as a group. But the system could provide residents with the opportunity to meet and support each other as a group – to get to know each other and to talk over how their care is run. This depends very much on the training and attitude of the key worker, to act as an informal leader, but it is an option that could be worth trying out in Homes where a key worker system is well established.

Residents' committees

Where residents are able to take part in discussions, their contributions can be very valuable in the running of a Home, and they are a way of helping people feel their advice is worth something. Residents can be very effective – and can recommend quite important changes in the way a Home is run. If you do have some residents who can form the nucleus of a committee and it is not something you have considered, put the idea to them. It can be very important for this kind of group to meet perhaps once a month.

Manager 'We used to have a residents' committee, but unfortunately the people on that committee are no longer with us, and we don't have anyone at present who can take it on. But we do have a meeting which one of the senior staff leads. They talk about anything they have problems with – sometimes it's to do with other residents. Changes in the menu is what they always like to talk about. We discuss where to go on outings and events – and before we redecorated two lounges we discussed the paints and wallpapers. Things like that to help them to be involved.'

Relatives' support groups

Meetings may be useful not just for residents, but for their relatives too. Often they have mixed feelings about their relations being in a Home. They may feel guilty, they may be concerned that the Home provides proper care, and they may want to make sure that they get value for money. Relatives' meetings give a chance to bring these issues into the open. It is obviously very important how the meeting is chaired. If no resident is able or willing to take it on, the chair will need sound skills in running this kind of meeting.

KEY POINTS

- Are there always people coming in and out of the Home?
- Do you know the names of regular visitors?
- Are care staff trained to bring visitors a pot of tea or coffee? Make sure facilities are readily available.
- How many residents have very weak arms or legs and might benefit from help in strengthening them?
- Do you have an occasional or regular visiting choir? Do the residents join in with the singing, or just sit and listen?

- Are there personal services such as hairdressing, paid or voluntary, which help residents to improve their appearance?

- Are some members of your staff trained to lead a reminiscence group?

- Do you encourage new residents to bring books with them to the Home?

- Do you have a special arrangement with a local library for borrowing books?

- Are you on the mailing list for publishers of large print books?

- Are there enough small seating areas in the Home for residents to meet and talk together in small groups?

- If you have key workers, do their residents ever meet together as a small group for mutual support?

- Are residents involved in the choice of menu?

QUALITY CONTROL

Social Services team leader 'We are now entering a quality era. We have been through other eras in the past, but now the public has greater expectations of public services. This includes the independent and voluntary sector, and places a great responsibility on them to provide the quality that the public demands. It has major implications across the residential sectors, because the quality services will survive, and those places that cannot provide a quality service will go under.'

Strong words, and ones that managers would be wise not to ignore. As outlined in the Introduction, inspection units for residential homes are now established in every local authority. Units work to guidelines issued by the Department of Health to make sure that residential homes (except those exempt because of having Crown Immunity) in the area are regularly inspected and monitored. The guidelines are not prescriptive, and the practices between one authority and another may be different. Inspection units are responsible to the director of social services in each authority, but they operate independently from the social services divisions responsible for providing or managing care.

The inspection unit

Policy Guidance for *Community Care in the Next Decade and Beyond.* 'Inspection is a process of external examination intended to establish whether a service is being managed and provided in conformity with expected standards . . . . Inspection supports, but is not a substitute for, good management. The responsibility for ensuring delivery of services of the right quality and for monitoring outcomes rests primarily with those commissioning the service.'

As explained throughout the book, managers of Homes in all sectors, including local authority homes, are answerable to the inspection unit. If privately managed homes have a contract with the local authority to provide care, they will also have to conform with the requirements of the purchaser of care, ie the social services department.

Units will focus on inspection of residential care in the public, private and voluntary sectors, and on the registration of private and voluntary care homes. They will evaluate the quality of care provided and the quality of life experienced in residential care homes. Each unit will aim at making sure that the care is consistent for Homes in their area and will respond to demands for quality control.

Support from the inspectorate

The Department of Health practice guidance recognises that individual Homes will need support and encouragement to bring, or keep, their services up to standard. The kind of support will differ in individual authorities and forms part of the inspection process. The inspectors will make allowance for the type of resident to be catered for. Every year there has to be one planned inspection, which takes at least a day, and one unplanned inspection, where inspectors may focus on talking to residents or staff and of which owners are not given advance notice.

Principal Inspector 'At the annual inspection we first confirm that registration details are absolutely right – for instance, a proprietor may have moved out of the Home to a private address. Then we check the numbers of residents, their dependency levels and their ages, because this links up with minimum staffing levels. We look at residents' health care, social care – contacts outside the Home, including relative's religious needs and general quality of life.

'Then we inspect the Home itself – the physical environment, the actual rooms registered, facilities like lifts, the state of the Home as regards decor, cleanliness and odour, wall covering, furniture. We check for any repairs or maintenance that should be carried out.'

In addition, inspections include checks on fire and safety standards, heating, lighting and laundry, the catering side – times of meals, the availability of choice, special diets, etc. Finally, the inspection takes a close look at management, staffing, including staff training, records and complaints.

Principal Inspector 'We make out a very detailed inspection report covering all these aspects, and we summarise all the points requiring action with a time scale of two months, six months or twelve months. Each report is sent to the proprietor for completion, so that they confirm the action they must take. Every inspection, announced or unannounced will have such a report.'

Annual reports

Every inspection unit will have to publish an annual report which is available to the public. This will provide information about individual Homes and other services for use by those placing contracts. The report might include:

An analysis of aggregate staffing arrangements.

Staff workload and areas of activity.

Residents' ages and dependency profiles.

A summary of the outcome of an inspection,
including quality of care and recommendations.

Individual Homes or other services may be identified in the report – the only exceptions will be for legal reasons – and there will be public access, subject to legal advice, to reports or summaries of reports on individual Homes.

Objections to inspectorate reports can be made through the complaints procedure systems which are in force in local authorities.

Advisory committees

The social services department in every local authority has to appoint an advisory committee to the inspection unit, without executive powers. This acts as a forum for exchange of views and mutual support between registration authority officers and any service providers who are subject to inspection or quality control. Advisory committees have a number of functions:

To comment on annual and other reports.

To advise on development of self-assessment.

To review performance and training.

To promote mutual understanding and good working relationships between the unit and service providers.

Individual Home owners and managers are represented on the advisory committee and should make sure that their views and problems are given a proper hearing through those representatives.

KEY POINTS

- The NHS and Community Care Act, 1990 should lead to improvements in the quality of care expected and how it is monitored.
- Homes in every sector will be subject to regular inspections.
- The public will have access to the inspectorate's reports on individual Homes, through a set procedure.

WORKING WITH THE INSPECTORATE

Owners and managers are well advised to be open and co-operative with inspection visits. This will help to ensure a good quality of care and has the advantage of making sure their Homes come out well in reports. Their future business will depend on them. The responsibility of providing quality may be particularly hard for owner/managers of small Homes, which operate a small profit margin and already have to make difficult choices about the care they provide. So it is important at this stage to think again about your aims and objectives in running the Home.

Monitoring your performance

How you perform as a manager is linked with your own development as a person – this is what research into management performance suggests. It means that if you have thought out your own personal targets or priorities in life, then the people whom you lead will have a clear idea of what you expect. Self-monitoring, like self-motivation, cannot be a set of woolly ideas, it needs clear thought and sometimes an honest answer to some difficult questions.

At some stage, you will have drawn up a statement of the aims and objectives of your Home. Have you drawn up a similar set of personal goals for yourself, and do they coincide with those for the Home? Be honest! They could be along the following lines:

- What do I want to get out of managing this Home? Is it to make money, to enjoy power, a desire to help others and to use my skills in care? Is there a mixture of several motives?

- Am I using all my skills and talents in my work? If not, what is left out and can it be used?

- What management skills am I weak in and how can I change this?

- Do I get all the support I need? If not, how can I obtain it?

- Am I able to ask the people who work for me to evaluate my performance?

- Do people work for me because they are afraid of me or because they share my goals?

- Do I look regularly at my targets to check whether I am achieving them?

Think carefully about each of these questions and answer them as honestly as you can. There are no right or wrong answers, but they may help you find out whether you are going where you want to in life.

Evaluating your staff

Many of the questions given above could also be asked of the people who work for you. When you talk to them about their work, keep their personal goals in mind too. Caring is, by its nature, an outgoing job, but it starts from within. It needs people who have warmth, a sense of humour and who like communicating with others. And people who give out those qualities need to have them recognised. Being good with an older person, giving them love or making them laugh are not extras to the job, they are part of it – and are as important as practical skills.

So keep your own personal goals and the personal needs of your staff in mind, as you consider ways of making sure your Home provides the service that the community increasingly requires.

Finding support

The checklist for monitoring your performance on page 143 may throw up some areas in your life or your working methods where you feel you need support. There are several ways you should be able to find this. Many of them have been mentioned earlier in the book, but a summary is given below on four key areas of support:

- from impartial advice
- in liaison with the inspection unit
- by linking up with other Home managers
- from trade unions

Impartial advice

An advisory committee for a Home could have a brief which is much the same as that for the local authority advisory committee. Such a committee can act as a window into community needs and also advise on problem areas of management and finance.

Government agencies offer free consultancy sessions and booklets for new and growing businesses which may be able to offer help in broad areas. For detailed advice which is tailored to your own business, you should be able to get first-class help through a Training and Enterprise Council (see p 165).

A firm of accountants may prove to be a good investment where it looks as if a Home is heading for financial difficulties and a radical look at the financial management is required. Such advice is not cheap, and as a manager you will need to balance the expense against the alternatives, such as getting into debt or going out of business.

Inspection unit

The inspection unit can help and advise managers of Homes about how to improve care. They are not there to put Homes out of business. So you should expect a positive response from the inspectorate if you consult them.

Ask their advice at an early stage if you plan any changes to your buildings, the type of care you offer or if you want to move into a different market. The inspection units will contain staff with a variety of skills, including special consultants on short-term secondments, so they should be able to provide a fresh eye on the care scene.

Links with other managers

It is always helpful to find support from people in the same position as yourself. The addresses of professional associations for owners and managers of private residential homes are given on page 164, and they will be all too familiar with problems facing owners and managers. Most of these organisations have national and regional sections. The regional officers will have particular knowledge of your area, and will be developing their own links with inspectorates, etc, which you could find valuable.

On an informal basis, a group of Homes may pool its resources in areas such as training. This is common in the voluntary sector, where one housing association or trust runs a number of Homes. So if, for example, you decide to set up a day course on first aid or continence management, you could invite staff from nearby Homes to take part on the assumption that your staff will be invited to similar courses which they run. This co-operation could be extended to events or care – for instance, having residents from two Homes going on a trip which will fill a coach, rather than having two separate outings.

Finally, if you work on your own, you may like to consider bringing together other similarly placed owner/managers to pool ideas and problems on a more formal basis. The large Homes and the new consortia which may be buying into ex-local authority homes will have much greater resources than a single Home owner. It makes sense to have access to a larger group.

Help from trade unions

The role of the unions is increasingly important in maintaining the quality of care. All local authorities recognise trade unions, and their members get support on a number of professional issues which include regular newsletters which discuss issues such as new thinking on care provision, medical or nursing news, training schemes and so on. Trade unions may well have something to offer Homes in the private sector, and it is worth inviting a local leader to discuss some of things which are faced not only by yourself but by people working at all levels in residential care.

Your attitude and goals

While all the support systems mentioned above may offer help and advice, they are, like the inspectorate itself, 'arms length' supporters. Owners and managers themselves have the final responsibility for making sure that quality care is provided, based on the guidelines suggested elsewhere in the book. But the most important part of giving quality of care comes from your own attitude to your work and your own goals in life.

The next few years will provide great challenges for everyone who offers residential care for older people. There will be pressure to keep costs down, but there will also be pressure to offer a quality product. How you balance these two will depend on the support you ask for and get, on your willingness to make changes and on your professional skills and personal qualities as a manager.

KEY POINTS

- Get to know and talk to your local inspectorate.
- Check out their particular areas of expertise.
- Before an inspection is due, arrange an informal visit so that you can discuss any changes that could be made before a formal inspection.
- Are you a member of a professional association for care homes?
- Do you know other Home managers in your area and use them as a source of support?
- Have you ever arranged a joint event or training session with them?
- What would be the problems and benefits of a joint venture?
- Have you ever discussed such a move with your staff?
- How do you keep costs down and continue to offer a quality product?

Branching Out

As residential homes develop the quality of care which they offer, many managers will be looking at ways to offer that expertise to a wider community. One of the implications of the NHS and Community Care Act 1990 is that local authorities will move towards being purchasers rather than direct providers of care. It is also likely that local authorities will look to the independent sector to provide services which up to now have been available mainly from social services departments.

So in the future there may be opportunities for growth which forward looking managers will want to exploit. Their Homes may have an opportunity to offer a number of specialist services, such as:

- short-term care
- day care facilities
- special activities and events
- care and meals for people in their own homes
- a resource centre for information, services and equipment
- a 'bed availability' scheme

It is as well to remember that spreading the care net too wide can have its dangers – for management, for permanent staff and for the residents. This chapter explores both these aspects of moving into different areas of care.

LIAISING WITH THE LOCAL COMMUNITY

As a Home manager, you already keep in contact with a number of people and authorities. As community care develops and changes over the next few years, these contacts may take up more of your time, and it will be more important than ever to make and maintain good links with your local community. This will help you maintain an adequate number of residents and also keep your Home in mind when new facilities are sought.

Personal recommendation is always important to a Home manager. Ambassadors for your Home could be your advisory committee, members of a resident's family and friends as well as the people who visit the Home in an official capacity. They may have considerable influence on where prospective residents are placed. It is worth making a serious effort to get to know all these different people, and to be willing to ask and take advice. This will help your business as well as provide for better care.

As we emphasise throughout the text, you should always welcome visitors to the Home. Managing a Home which is welcoming does not just happen, it has to be planned. All staff have to be included if an atmosphere of an 'open establishment' is to prevail. You may also want to designate one member of staff for a set shift to be responsible for visitors. A private space for talking with visitors is also important.

People who visit the Home will, of course, include professionals (GPs, district/community nurses, physiotherapists, etc) as well as relatives, friends and potential residents. Making an effort to get to know professionals over a cup of coffee is likely to help your business relationship. It also helps to visit them in their place of work. The subject of working with local services is covered in detail in the chapter 'Managing A Home'

An advisory council or governing board

Governing bodies and the appointment of trustees are common practice in voluntary homes, and under the Charities Act 1960 the appointment of trustees carries legal responsibilities and duties. Other Homes may have an advisory group drawn from the community which is sympathetic to the aims of the Home. Either way, managers find these groups a useful source of support and advice.

Where there is a formal body which advises or directs the affairs of a Home, you will probably, as manager, be expected to present facts and figures at a board meeting and talk them through at regular intervals. It could include the yearly accounts or a budget for a particular project or a projection of income needs for the next twelve months. The meeting would then have a chance to look at all the figures to see whether they were viable and to suggest alternatives. These meetings also give a manager the chance to raise matters where a fresh viewpoint may help solve a difficult problem. This could be matters to do with staffing, care or marketing, finding new clients.

Informal advisory bodies may not make binding recommendations, but their suggestions can be extremely valuable. If you do decide to set up your own group, suitable members could include:

–   a local business person, who can give business advice;

    someone who understands the conditions of old age and who will act as an advocate to the residents;

–   a representative from the staff;

    someone with contacts in the social services department;

–   someone from the medical or nursing professions.

Offering short-term care

Short-term care provided to older people for a week or two can serve several different purposes. It may be used as a means of introducing someone to residential care with a view to a long-term placement. It may be an opportunity for someone who lives alone to have a break, meet other people and have an improved diet. In this way, periods of regular short-stay may enable an older person to continue to live in their own home with opportunities for occasional support and rehabilitation.

The majority of older people in need of care are not in a residential home but remain in their own home, looked after by a private, unsalaried carer who is usually a close relation. The stress this places on the carer – who has sometimes to be available twenty-four hours on duty – is well-documented.

Respite care or short-stay means just that – the elderly person comes to stay in a residential home for a short period to give the carer a respite from the

punishing daily round. It also provides a new outlook for the person, per
haps the chance to meet new people and have more stimulation than they get
at home. Residential homes also provide respite care as a half-way house
between hospital and home, where a person requires care rather than nursing.

Owner 'I have someone here for a couple of months who has been very ill. And
there's a little lady who came here from hospital after a cataract operation.
She's going home on Saturday. I like to keep a couple of rooms for short-
term care. I feel it brings something new into the Home.'

Recent research into the use of short-stay and respite care has shown that it
can create difficulties of disorientation and make an older person more confused. These effects can be minimised by good assessment, admission and
review procedures. The use of a key worker can also help someone settle
during the transition to a residential care setting. It is important to make sure
that the system is working efficiently and that long-term residents in the
Home are not affected by people who only come for a short time.

Managers who are considering short-term care as an option need to have
clear objectives, which should include:
– the purpose of a short-term stay;
– the criteria for admission;
– a review procedure.

Day care facilities

It is quite usual to find day care facilities attached to a local authority home.
Usually the rooms for day care are separate from the residential side of the
Home even though the people from the community use the Home's catering
facilities. A small day centre could be an option for a residential home, with
elderly people from the local neighbourhood coming in for the day.

You will need to consider all the implications of this very carefully. Ask
yourself the following questions:
– Are there sufficient public rooms, toilets and dining facilities?
– How many more staff would you need on the care and catering side?
– Day care people are generally more active than full-time residents. Can
  you offer enough for them to do?

- What effect would a day care facility have on the permanent residents? Would they feel dispossessed from the Home?
- Consider how welcome visitors feel at present when they visit the home? Would these new arrivals feel welcome or unwanted?

If you feel confident that you have the right staff, facilities and attitudes, organise a pilot scheme for a few weeks to see whether day care provision can work out in practice.

Special activities and events

Not so demanding as providing regular day care, your Home could still be the place where older people come for occasional days or for morning activities. It could be a weekly physiotherapy class, for which you provide the facilities, or a shopping expedition at a time set aside for older people in local shops, or a trip to a matinée. Other residential homes in your area might also be interested in suggesting the idea to some of their more active residents.

An alternative approach is to offer a venue for stroke rehabilitation for older people who still live in their own homes.

Home care for local people

Home helps or home care workers may, like porters, soon be a thing of the past, but the need for help has never been greater. There are of course agencies which provide services to people at home – at a price. A nursing agency has to employ properly qualified nurses, but an agency offering general home help can have any number of unqualified people on their books – from a foreign student half way round her world tour who needs cash for the next stage of her trip, to a capable mother of three who has returned to work outside her home. In other words, there is no consistency of quality and no guarantee from their background that the person knows much about caring for older people.

This is where a residential home could offer good home care from experienced, well-trained staff. It could suit former care assistants who would like the part-time work, but you would need to think it out very carefully. In the long term, most of the work would probably come via social services departments, and is not likely to be under consideration until after 1993.

However, it could be something you might try out as a private concern, if you are in an area where there are older people in need who could afford these services.

- Estimate how many staff hours you would need to cover twice-daily care for five elderly people?
- Do you have access to suitably trained staff, or could you find them?
- If staff came from an agency, what would the fee be?
- What would you need to charge to make a profit?
- Have you the office back-up to run a day care scheme?
- Would you be able to offer a meal prepared in your kitchen to people in the community, what would be the cost of providing meals and would this be profitable?

Becoming a service centre

Changes in the role of residential homes in countries outside Britain, notably Germany, Denmark and the United States, have been under discussion for a number of years. The changing role is about a residential home becoming a 'service centre' or 'social shop' offering a range of services to older people in the community. It is an idea which smaller Homes in the UK could only respond to in a limited way, but which offers potential for development especially in the voluntary sector and local authority homes.

One German residential home has accommodation for over 150 people, and in addition offers the following community services:

- a daily lunch service with a cafeteria system;
- facilities for running courses in pre-retirement education preparation for old age and living in residential care;
- day care for those requiring nursing attention;
- an office base for the local area social work team;
- special facilities, such as a gymnasium or a hydrotherapy pool;
- equipment for loan, such as wheelchairs, walking frames, eating or sewing aids for disabled people;
- music, shows and exhibitions;
- a free bi-monthly newspaper for 3,000 local elderly people;
- rooms to let for public hire.

In Britain, there have not so far been any establishments able to operate on such a large scale. However, some Homes have been adapted and are now resource centres for all kinds of services for older people, such as nursing, health visiting, physiotherapy, occupational therapy, chiropody and dental care. Other homes open up their buildings to the community with perhaps a bar, a leisure centre, laundry facilities and so on. As mentioned earlier, some Homes are offering short-term stay for people, intermittent respite beds and forms of rotational or shared care.

The idea of a residential home acting as a service centre is a major new development in the provision of care. Such a centre could provide not only services, but also training and research into health care in old age. And, for private sector owners and care staff, a service centre would provide the opportunity to meet, socialise, take further training and exchange ideas.

Such developments are being studied by a series of demonstration projects set up under the Department of Health 'Caring in Homes Initiative', which is following up recommendations of the Wagner Report *Residential Care: A Positive Choice*. The Caring in Homes Initiative is concerned with improving the quality of residential care and ensuring that residence is a positive choice. It has highlighted the need for more service flexibility, more choice and a greater understanding of people's needs.

The 'Window in Homes' programme as part of this action-research work is focusing on the importance of links between residential homes and the community. Good establishments are naturally integrated into the local community with effective networks. The location and the size of a Home will be important, as well as the services it provides. The concept of a resource centre which brings together a range of services is likely to have an important part to play in the future development of community care.

Drawbacks of branching out

Many of the suggestions outlined above have been based on the assumption that more care will be required in the community and that local authorities will be a major purchaser. However, many authorities have not yet published their community care plans, or have not even formulated their policies. While managements should be aware of what they might be asked to provide, it would clearly not be prudent to assume this provision without the offer of a well-thought-out contract.

At this stage, managers would be best to consider some of the less expensive options and carry out careful financial planning into the pitfalls of over-extension which has proved to be a way to bankruptcy for a number of seemingly profitable enterprises.

Managers should not underestimate the effect of even minor changes on the nature of the Home. After all, residents are encouraged to think of it as their home. Suddenly there would be a whole lot of strangers, often fitter and stronger, wandering around, perhaps sitting in residents' chairs, demanding attention from care assistants and wanting to make changes in routines – all things that some older people find upsetting.

The staff too could find their working day disrupted by branching out. They have got to know the permanent residents and established close relationships with them. In an extended Home their focus of attention may be shifted. A floating number of non-permanent people in receipt of care could cause all kinds of tensions which have not been foreseen.

KEY POINTS

- Do you have a room which is under used where classes could be held?

- Have you approached other Home managers about formal or informal links?

- How many demands would such a scheme make on your own time and that of your staff?

- The possibilities for extending care provision are not likely to be clarified until local authority care plans are published.

- Bringing older people into a residential home for day care or special activities may upset many permanent residents and also the care staff.

- Managers should look at the opportunities, but are advised to proceed with caution.

Training and Staff Development

Good intentions are never a substitute for good training for staff and for management. Many of the difficulties experienced in Homes occur because those in charge are not aware either of the importance of making sure everyone knows what to do or of the training opportunities now available. In this chapter we give suggestions on how managers and their staff may develop and improve their skills, which includes working for National Vocational Qualifications.

In addition there is information about induction courses, supervised work place training and courses which staff can attend on day-release from the Home. We also cover staff development programmes, City and Guilds and BTEC courses, training and specialist packs.

STAFF TRAINING

Under the inspection system set up by the NHS and Community Care Act, 1990, managers are expected to make sure that their staff are properly trained in all aspects of their work and this is an important area which the inspectors will check carefully.

Some care assistants may already have had some form of training in care when they are appointed to a post, but others often have experience of working with elderly people with no formal qualifications. Any newly recruited care, catering or domestic staff should have their training needs identified as soon as possible, a process which starts at the interview. Although they can have training on the premises as soon as they start their new job, many also attend a local college of further education and other training centres through a day-release scheme.

An effective approach to training should include all staff in the Home, whether members of the caring, administrative or management teams. There should be clear statements on the mission and objectives of the Home, and all staff should be assessed to determine their specific needs to meet these objectives. The training programme should be regularly revised and reviewed to make sure it is keeping in step with any new requirements or changes in policy of the Home.

The induction course

Every Home has by law to provide an induction programme for new staff, which usually includes the provision of an induction or information pack and special training sessions. The induction pack contains all the information about the Home which will be useful. A typical pack will include:

— Aims or philosophy of the Home.

— Profile of the residents.

— Map of the buildings.

— List of regular meetings.

— Staff member's: job description; duty sheets (including special tasks for each shift); conditions of service (grievance and complaints procedure) and a statement about confidentiality.

— Health and safety at work regulations.

— Fire regulations.

— Food hygiene regulations.

— The resident's: rights in the Home; admission/review documents; accident forms; assessment and reporting forms; sample care plan and evaluation sheet.

The induction pack may also include information on trade unions and any particular details about the Home.

On arrival

The induction programme is carried out by the manager or a senior member of staff, who meet the new care assistant for a regular period once or twice a week. They go through the pack, and discuss all aspects of care, so that by the end the care assistant is thoroughly familiar with all aspects of the job.

How staff are trained in the early days often depends on the size of the Home, but this is a crucial time for the new arrival. Managers should provide support and supervision at all times. The new assistant should be encouraged to speak up at meetings, to ask for help or advice, and the manager should make a point of talking to them informally about the job or any problems they face. The book *Taking Good Care*, also published by Age Concern England, has a more detailed discussion about the first days of work (see page 176 for ordering).

New domestic and catering staff may not need such a detailed induction programme, but they should also have regular meetings with a senior staff member. Their induction programme should emphasise:

The aims and philosophy of the Home.

How to relate to older people.

An appropriate diet for older people.

The importance of good hygiene in the Home.

Fire, health and safety and food regulations.

Laundry and cleaning methods.

The proper disposal of waste.

Dealing with emergencies.

A mentor

Often an experienced carer acts as mentor during the induction period – someone who knows the duties, knows which residents need special care and may demand attention or like to be involved in the Home's activities. The mentor is also best placed to find out more about the new care assistant, their interests and talents, and be able to involve them in the life of the Home. In large Homes, a mentor scheme is particularly valuable. One of the most common difficulties faced by new staff is a feeling of isolation, that they are not one of the 'family'.

Review of training

It is important that senior staff supervise and observe new staff at work, so that any areas in which they may be weak, such as communication skills, can also be brought into the induction training, as well as highlighted for further sessions. Feedback – showing staff that you see and appreciate what they are doing, or giving them constructive criticism – is essential at this time. The following questions will help you check your training provision:

- Do you have an induction programme, including an information pack, for new staff?

- Have you revised or checked it recently to cover new practices and regulations?

- Have you tried a mentoring system?

- How much do you find out about new members of staff when they join the Home?

- Do you ask the residents for their views on new staff?

- Do you give new staff regular feedback on their progress?

Once staff are established in their duties, there are several ways in which managers can arrange to develop their skills.

They could arrange for experienced and suitably qualified senior staff to supervise the work place training of newer assistants. Special training sessions in the Home for some or all staff also help to improve the quality of care they can give.

Managers should also be aware of training opportunities away from the Home, which may be day release at a local college of further education or in-service courses run by organisations such as Age Concern England. All these types of training may be part of a National Vocational Qualification (NVQ) or existing vocational qualification.

National Vocational Qualifications

These qualifications are being introduced into all areas of working life and involve assessing people on their ability to carry out a particular task or range of associated tasks. This takes into account their current position and gives credit for their prior knowledge and skills. Ideally this is carried out by supervisors, who have themselves been accredited to assess staff in this way. Staff need to demonstrate that they are competent, and have the appropriate knowledge to carry out the task effectively. This is an area where further training may be necessary.

The NVQs are graded into levels from I to VII, which move from manual work through to management. It is a very large undertaking which will take some time to complete. At the present time the Residential, Domiciliary and Day Care Competencies are being converted into specific NVQs which can then be gained by staff working in those areas. There are also NVQs in domestic and catering work. These are all at levels II and III.

It is likely that in the future all qualifications and certificates offered by examining bodies will be designated to a particular NVQ level, though for some time both systems are likely to run in parallel. For example, the City and Guilds 325.1, Community Care Practice, is the usual qualification for care assistants. There is now an equivalent NVQ at level II and both will be available for some time.

Training for management

Much of the current training is based on new research into how to provide the best care for older people. Managers as well as staff will benefit from going on training courses.

There are many courses which are specifically designed for management. On the business side, local colleges and polytechnics run courses which cover all aspects of running a business, such as bookkeeping and finance, strategic planning, office administration, leadership and interpersonal skills, working with a team and so on.

There are also care-related courses, which can be taken on site or away from the workplace. Obviously an owner/manager will not be able to take much time off from the actual running of a Home, but all further training should lead to greater efficiency and cost effectiveness. It cannot be stressed too much how important it is for managers to take time to further their own professional development as well as encouraging that of their staff.

The Department of Employment has now published a set of management standards which link management skills with the top end of the National Vocational Qualifications. There are two levels: Management Competence I and II, which are designed to cover a wide variety of occupations and which are transferable between occupations. Many training organisations now incorporate them.

The key purpose for both levels is 'to achieve the organisation's objectives and continuously improve its performance'. The following are the key roles, which have two associated units of competence: managing operations, managing finance, managing people and managing information.

Managers are able to obtain an MCI endorsed Certificate Level Management Award, which will be recommended to the National Council for Vocational Qualifications (NCVQ) as above level IV in their hierarchy.

KEY POINTS

- Local authority inspection units and some of the professional associations listed on page 164 will monitor training programmes. This is part of the registration and inspection process.
- Regular training for all staff should be part of everyone's work schedules.

STAFF DEVELOPMENT PROGRAMMES

There are several kinds of training which managers can arrange for themselves and their staff to be carried out in the Home and incorporated into an NVQ.

For example, senior members of staff can hold regular training sessions on topics in which they have expertise. These may cover a range of care or domestic duties such as fire drills, working with groups, diet for older people, lifting techniques, etc.

As mentioned throughout the text, training can also be provided by an outside expert, such as a physiotherapist, a district nurse or occupational therapist in specific care related to their disciplines. This kind of training is an important part of a therapist's job, and can be a valuable source of support for a manager.

The distance learning packages listed on pages 162–163 provide a full training programme including group leader's material and worksheets, etc for trainees. These courses are comprehensive and cover a wide range of important topics.

In-house training offered by an outside organisation is becoming increasingly popular with managers. Courses are tailored for each particular Home or group of Homes in one area both by national organisations, such as Age Concern England, or locally, often from a college of further education.

City and Guilds courses

These cover all branches of care, including care of older people, and they provide a good foundation for later specialisation in this area. Courses may be taken on day-release, part-time or full-time. They are:

- 356 Practical Caring Skills PI and PII
- 331 Family and Community Care
- 325.1 Community Care Practice
- 325.2 Foundation Management for Care
- 325.3 Advanced Management for Care
- 706 Catering

The Management for Care courses are designed for owners, managers and supervisory staff from residential, domiciliary and day care institutions. The minimum age is usually 20 years, and candidates should have at least two junior members of staff working with them. The courses involve over 200 hours, through day release and evening work. There is a mix of learning methods, including working with a group and independently.

Other courses

There is a BTEC 1st Diploma course for care assistants which provides basic training for those who wish to pursue a career in the care field. At present there is a CCETSW course being run for people in the social services as an update, but this particular course is under review at the present moment, and is likely to be discontinued.

Food handling courses are available at the Royal Society of Health, the Institute of Environmental Health Officers and The Royal Institute of Public Health and Hygiene.

Training packs and initiatives

Small Business Programme
*Management development for the growing
business, prepared by the Open University and
Cranfield School of Management, offered widely
through local colleges.*

Cranfield School
of Management
Institute of Technology
Cranfield
Bedford MK43 0AL
Tel: 0234 750111

Training for Care
*A package covering a wide range of topics of
interest to staff working in homes for older people.
There is special material for group leaders and
participants.*

Local Government
Management Board
Arndale Centre, Luton
Bedford LU1 2TS
Tel: 0582 451166

SCROLL (Social Care Open Learning Project)
*A pack containing a series of booklets on social
care, first published by the Cranfield Institute of
Technology.*

Arta Ltd
123 Lichfield Grove
Finchley
London N3 2JL
Tel: 081-343 4833

Training Support Programme
*This is a Department of Health initiative which
provides funds for training to local authorities and
may also involve residential care staff from the
private and voluntary sectors.*

Details from:
Your social services
training department

Specialist packs

According to Need
*A video and trainer's guide on the cultural needs
of older people from ethnic minorities.*

Age Concern Training
(South Region)
Age Concern England
Address on page 174

Age Exchange Reminiscence Boxes
A set of boxes covering events from earlier in the century (childhood games, going shopping, World War II, school days, etc).

Age Exchange
The Reminiscence
Centre
11 Blackheath Village
London SE3 9LA
Tel: 081-318 9105

Exercising the Imagination
Games and exercises for fun and stimulation.

Institute of
Social Inventions
20 Heber Road
London NW2 6AA

Golden Opportunities Part 2
A pack with video, trainers' notes, assessment guide and the book Reminiscence with Elderly People.

Pavilion Publishing
47 Landsdown Place
Hove
East Sussex BN3 1HH
Tel: 0273 821650

Living, Loving and Ageing
A video on sexual and personal relationships in later life.

Age Concern England
Address on page 174

Safe and Secure
How to deal with potential violence at work.

Outset Publishing, Unit 8
Conqueror Industrial
Estate
Moonhurst Road
St Leonard's on Sea
East Sussex TN38 3NA
Tel: 0424 854124

Using Reminiscence
A training pack with tape/slide, video and manual to encourage the promotion of good practice for professionals and non-professionals.

Help the Aged
16/18 St James's Walk
London EC1R 0BE
Tel: 071-253 0253

Further Information

USEFUL ADDRESSES

Professional associations

These associations provide advice and information for managers of private residential homes. (MARCH is for managers in all sectors.)

National Care Homes Association
A confederation of local associations throughout the UK, whose principal aim is to lobby the government for the benefit of residents in care homes. The association is self-monitoring, and all Homes applying for membership are inspected.

5 Bloomsbury Place
London WC1A 2QA
Tel: 071-436 1871

British Federation of Care Home Proprietors
A federation with committees in 14 regions throughout the country. After application, every Home is inspected by an independent inspector to make sure it comes up to the standards for membership.

852 Melton Road
Thurmaston
Leicester LE4 8BN
Tel: 0533 640095

National Association for Mental After-Care in Registered Care Homes (MARCH)
An association of care homes in all sectors which offer care to people who suffer from mental illness or dementia. Operates a bed vacancy service with quality assurance. Homes are inspected prior to membership.

c/o Heathercroft Services
2A Cornfield Lane
Eastbourne BN21 4NE
Tel: 0323 645408

Social Care Association
The association promotes good practice in care,
provides training and support, undertakes research
and offers consultancy, advice and information.

23a Victoria Road
Surbiton
Surrey KT6 4JZ
Tel: 081-390 6832

Sources of business advice

The following organisations provide advice and help about setting up, running or expanding a business.

Rural Development Commission Business Service
For advice and loans for businesses to be
developed in rural England.

141 Castle Street
Salisbury SP1 3TP
Tel: 0722 336255

Training and Enterprise Councils (TECS)
Regionally based in the UK to advise businesses
setting up in their area. Ring Freephone number
for your nearest TEC.

For London
Freephone 0800 222 999
For rest of UK
Freephone 0800 444 246

Local authority incentives
These operate throughout England to develop
business in inner city areas.

Your local authority
will advise you about
the address of your
nearest unit.

Scottish Enterprise Agency
For help in setting up a business in Scotland. Has
13 regional offices.

120 Bothwell Street
Glasgow G2 7JP
Tel: 041-248 2700

Local Chambers of Commerce
These comprise members from all areas of local
business to share advice and information.

Look in your local
telephone directory for
the address.

National Federation of Self-Employed and Small Businesses
Acts as a pressure group for small businesses
and people who are self-employed. Also supplies
to members an information pack on setting up in
business.

32 St Anne's Road West
Lytham St Annes
Lancs FY8 1NY

Alliance of Small Firms and Self-Employed People (ASP)
Offers an enquiry service to members on a range
of tax, legal and employment matters.

The Green
Calne
Wiltshire SN11 8DJ

Other useful organisations

Throughout the book we have referred to a number of organisations as a useful source of further information. Some of these have local groups, but we have included national addresses as a central source.

Age Concern Insurance Services
Orbital House
85–87 Croydon Road
Caterham
Surrey CR3 5YZ

Age Concern Training
PO Box B 96, Hammonds Yard
King Street
Huddersfield HD1 1WT

Alzheimer's Disease Society
3rd Floor
Bank Building
Fulham Broadway
London SW6 1EP

Arthritis Care
5 Grosvenor Crescent
London SW1X 7ER

BAHOH (British Association for the Hard of Hearing)
7–11 Armstrong Road
London W3 7JL

BASE (British Association for Service to the Elderly)
119 Hassell Street
Newcastle Under Lyme
Staffordshire ST5 1AX

CCETSW (Central Council for Education and Training in Social Work)
4th Floor
Derbyshire House
St Chad's Street
London WC1H 8AD

Centre for Policy on Ageing
25–31 Ironmonger Row
London EC1V 3QP

City and Guilds of London Institute
326 City Road
London EC1V 2PT

Communilink
4 Woodstock Road
London NW11 8ER

Continence Advisory Service
c/o Disabled Living Foundation
380–384 Harrow Road
London W9 2HU

Court of Protection
Stewart House
24 Kingsway
London WC2B 6HD

Disabled Living Foundation
380–384 Harrow Road
London W9 2HU

EXTEND (Exercise Training for the Elderly and/or Disabled)
1 The Boulevard
Sheringham
Norfolk N26 8LJ

Industrial Society
3 Carlton Terrace
London SW1Y 5DG

Institute of Complementary Medicine
PO Box 194
London SE16 1QZ

Institute of Environmental Health Officers
Chadwick House
London SE1 0QT

MIND (National Association for Mental Health)
22 Harley Street
London W1N 2ED

National Extension College
18 Brooklands Avenue
Cambridge CB2 2HN

The Open College
Carrera House
Villiers Street
London WC2N 6NN

Partially Sighted Society
Dean Clarke House
Southernhay East
Exeter EX1 1PE

RADAR (Royal Association for Disability and Rehabilitation)
25 Mortimer Street
London W1N 8AB

Royal Institute of Public Health and Hygiene
28 Portland Place
London W1N 4DE

RNIB (Royal National Institute for the Blind)
224 Great Portland Street
London W1N 6AA

RNID (Royal National Institute for the Deaf)
105 Gower Street
London WC1 6AH

Royal Society of Health
Royal Society House
38a St George's Drive
London SW1V 4BN

Scottish Action on Dementia
33 Castle Street
Edinburgh EH7 3DN

Talking Books RNIB Service
Mount Pleasant
Wembley
Middlesex HA0 1RR

Tower Printers
The Lodge
Haddington
York YO1 5DX

Winslow Press
Telford Road
Bicester
Oxon OX6 0TS

RECOMMENDED READING

Listed below are a number of useful books which your local library will be able to help you find. Alternatively you may want to buy one of these publications and could ask a local bookshop to order it.

Assessment Systems and Community Care Social Information Systems Ltd (HMSO, 1991)

Assessing Elderly People for Residential Care: A Practical Guide by June Neil. (National Institute of Social Work, 1989)

Coping with Caring: A Guide to Identifying and Supporting an Elderly Person with Dementia by Dr Brian Lodge. (MIND, 1981)

Creative Activities: An Activity Organiser's Handbook by Janette Fawdry and Betty Jackson. (Winslow Press, 1987)

Croner's Care Home Management, Croner Publications Ltd, Croner House, London Road, Kingston, Surrey KT2 6SR

Goal Planning with Elderly People by C Barrowclough and I Fleming. (Manchester University Press, 1986)

Group Work with the Elderly by Judith Hodgkinson. (Centre for Policy on Ageing, 1984, address on page 166)

Helping Older People: A Psychological Approach by Charles Twining, (John Wiley, 1988)

Home Life: A Code of Practice by Judith Hodgkinson. (Centre for Policy on Ageing, 1984, address on page 166)

Marketing for the Small Firm by Rick Brown. (Holt Rhinehart & Winston, 1985)

Management Skills in Social Care: A Handbook for Social Care Managers by John Harris and Des Kelly. (Gower Publications, 1991)

Nottingham Rehab Professional Catalogue, Nottingham Group, 17 Ludlow Hill Road, West Bridgford, Nottingham NG2 6HD

Reality Orientation: Principles and Practices (Manual) Una Holden et al. (Winslow Press, 1990)

Reminiscence with Elderly People by Andrew Norris. (Winslow Press, 1986)

Residential Care, A Positive Choice the Wagner Report (National Institute of Social Work/HMSO, 1988)

Rights in Residence Ed David Harris and Jim Hyland. (Social Care Association, 1989)

Staffing in Residential Care Homes Wagner Development Group. (National Institute of Social Work, 1990)

Starting Your Own Business Ed Edith Rudinger. (Consumers' Association and Hodder and Stoughton, 1990)

The Handbook on Oral History by Stephen Humphries. (Inter Action Imprint, 1984)

Validation Therapy by Naomi Feil. (Winslow Press, 1991)

Working with Dementia by Graham Stokes and Fiona Goudie. (Winslow Press, 1990)

Working in Residential Homes for Elderly People by C Paul Brearley. (Routledge, 1990)

The magazines listed below will help both managers and staff to keep up to date with issues affecting their work and information about new products and training opportunities.

- *Care Concern*
  Subscriptions Manager
  Hawker Publications Ltd
  13 Park House
  140 Battersea Park Road
  London SW11 4NB
  Tel: 071-720 2108

- *Community Care*
  Subscriptions Manager
  Oakfield House
  Pennymount Road
  Haywards Heath
  West Sussex RH16

- *Caring Times*
  Subscription Manager
  Hobson Publishing Plc
  Bateman Street
  Cambridge
  Tel: 0223 354551

- *Care Weekly*
  9 White Lion Street
  London N1 9XJ

- *This Caring Business*
  Carewell Publishing House
  1 St Thomas Road
  Hastings
  East Sussex TN34 3LG

- *National Carer*
  Subscription Manager
  London Leisure Publishing
  5 Bloomsbury Place
  London E4 7PU
  Tel: 081-524 6464

- *Reminiscence* (Newsletter)
  Help The Aged
  St James's Walk
  London EC1R 0BE
  Tel: 071-253 0253

APPENDIX

Appendix 1

CASHFLOW FORECAST   Business Name _____   Financial Year from _____ to _____

	Month		Month		Month		Month		Month		Month		Full Year Total	
	Budget	Actual	Budget	Actual	Budget	Actual	Budget	Actual	Budget	Actual	Budget	Actual	Budget	Actual
Sales														
Capital														
Other receipts														
Total inflow														
Expenses														
Salaries and wages for staff														
Tax and National Insurance														
Proprietor's/Partner's earnings														
Insurance premiums														
Subsistence														
Linen and household														
Medical and nursing aids														
Repairs and maintenance														
Capital equipment														
Electricity/gas/telephone														
Transport														
Special events														
Subscriptions														
Professional fees														
Contingency funds														
Total outflow														
Net inflow/(outflow)														
Cumulative I/(O)														

Appendix 2

A Programme for People Suffering from Dementia

First, you need to get a sense of a resident's overall level of orientation and disorientation, and particularly how well their sense of touch, smell, vision, hearing, taste and balance work.

Position yourself very close to the person so that they can see, hear and touch you easily. Make sure there is good lighting in the room. Do not even begin to communicate until you have established eye contact.

Body contact, such as holding someone's hand is a good way to help them realise that you are there, even when their eyes, thought and concentration wander. It will help them to focus on your presence better than if you keep a distance between the two of you.

Even if a person loses the train of a conversation or sentence, or gets their facts mixed up, you acknowledge the feeling behind the content.

For example, Mrs Simpson is talking about going home to visit her parents for dinner. You know that her parents are long since dead, but you do not need to hurt her by pointing that out, neither do you lie and say that they are alive. Instead you might say something like: 'It sounds to me like you miss your parents a lot, tell me something about them... are you more like your father or mother?... When you miss them, does it help to think about the nice times you had with them?'

Re-orient the resident as required, when there is a reason for doing so, or if they ask you. For example, if you must end a visit and bring the person to the dining room for their next meal, it is appropriate to say: 'It's nearly 12.00, lunch is ready, and I must go now, but I'll be back next week on Wednesday morning'. Or, if someone asks you: 'Where am I?' you should tell them, for example, 'You're in your room in Beech Grove'.

You must make sure, however, whether or not what the resident is really asking is: 'Where am I in this business of living my life?' If that is what they mean, then a appropriate answer might be: 'You are 85 years old, you've worked hard, had a family, the family is grown up now, and we are all proud that you have done so well. In spite of all the hard times, you always did the very best that you could and we love you for that.'

Give people lots of time to respond and repeat what you have just said if necessary. Never assume that the information given has been retained. Reaction and thinking time is significantly reduced in someone with dementia. Don't be embarrassed by long pauses.

Follow the 'thread' of the resident's conversation, and help them to maintain it when their memory is too weak to do so, or when there are distractions. For example, 'You were just telling me about....'

Try to collect reminiscence material for use in the Home. Reminisce liberally, and help the person to put things into the context of their own unique 'life story'.

Choose themes and subjects of conversation that are relevant to the person's interests, life, work and hobbies. Use props or 'triggers' to stimulate and prompt memory recall.

Be aware that intense reminiscing often evokes strong images, similar to those in dreaming and day dreaming states. When eyesight is decreased, a person may superimpose those 'inner images' onto a poorly perceived environment. This is not the same as hallucinating or crazy behaviour, so do not be perturbed by it.

from: 'Caregiving Approaches to Dementia' by Gemma Jones, published in *Holistic Health*, Spring 1989

Appendix 3

Management of Chronic Leg Ulcers

It is important that the type of ulcer is accurately diagnosed, and the initial diagnosis should be through taking blood pressure readings in the foot. In some health authorities, more specific scanning techniques for diagnosis are available. Residents with arterial leg ulcers may be referred for surgery, as these are harder to heal.

A typical symptom of a venous leg ulcer is a dark brown staining round the ulcer in the lower leg. Once the doctor has determined the nature of the ulcer, treatment is carried out by the district nurse, with the resident's help. A summary of the treatment suggested by the Department of Dermatology at the Slade Hospital, Oxford, is given below.

First, the nurse ensures that the wound is clean and applies a dressing. A new type of dressing, Granuflex Hydrocolloid, has been shown to speed up recovery both in leg ulcers, diabetic ulcers and pressure sores.

Next, the nurse puts a compression bandage on to the resident's leg at a time when it is least swollen – usually in the morning or after a 'legs up' period. The bandage should have 25–40 mm HG degrees of pressure at the ankle, reducing below the knee. Compression may be obtained by:

–   elastic bandages and external support bandages;

    paste bandages or Unna boots;

–   support stockings or Tubigrip.

A compression bandage should not impair the blood supply to the leg, but must provide adequate support.

Massage has also been found to improve venous and lymphatic drainage which will help to reduce the oedema and is recommended particularly when lymphatic drainage is impaired. As outlined on pages 71–72, residents can help greatly with the healing process by keeping the affected leg raised for regular periods during the day.

If after four to six weeks the healing of the venous ulcer is not progressing, the situation should be reviewed. It is important that exact measurements of the ulcer be made to assess progress. Where healing is difficult to achieve, the resident may have to be referred for hospital treatment.

About Age Concern

Good Care Management is one of a wide range of publications produced by Age Concern England – National Council on Ageing. In addition, Age Concern is actively engaged in training, information provision, research and campaigning for retired people and those who work with them. It is a registered charity dependent on public support for the continuation of its work.

Age Concern England links closely with Age Concern centres in Scotland, Wales and Northern Ireland to form a network of over 1,400 independent local UK groups. These groups, with the invaluable help of an estimated 250,000 volunteers, aim to improve the quality of life for older people and develop services appropriate to local needs and resources. These include advice and information, day care, visiting services, transport schemes, clubs, and specialist facilities for physically and mentally frail older people.

Age Concern England
1268 London Road
London SW16 4ER
Tel: 081-679 8000

Age Concern Scotland
54a Fountainbridge
Edinburgh EH3 9PT
Tel: 031-228 5656

Age Concern Wales
4th Floor
1 Cathedral Road
Cardiff CF1 9SD
Tel: 0222 371566

Age Concern Northern Ireland
6 Lower Crescent
Belfast BT7 1NR
Tel: 0232 245729

Publications from ◆◆◆ Books

A wide range of titles is published by Age Concern England under the ACE Books imprint

Health

In Control: Help with Incontinence
Penny Mares
Containing information about the nature and causes of incontinence and the sources of help available, this book has been written for anyone concerned about this problem, either professionally or at home. The text is illustrated throughout with drawings and case histories.
£4.50   0–86242–088–1

The Magic of Movement
Laura Mitchell
Full of encouragement, this book by TV personality Laura Mitchell is for those who are finding everyday activities more difficult. Includes gentle exercises to tone up the muscles and ideas to make you more independent and avoid boredom.
£3.95   0–86242–076–8

Know Your Medicines
Pat Blair
We would all like to know more about the medicines we take. The second edition of this successful guide is written for older people and their carers and examines how the body works and the effects of medication.
£6.95   0–86242–100–4

The Foot Care Book: An A-Z of fitter feet
Judith Kemp SRCh
A self-help guide for older people on routine foot care, this book includes an A–Z of problems, information on adapting and choosing shoes and a guide to who's who in foot care.
£2.95   0–86242–066–0

Money Matters

Your Rights

Sally West

A highly acclaimed annual guide to the State Benefits available to older people. Contains current information on Income Support, Housing Benefit and retirement pensions, among other matters, and provides advice on how to claim them.

Further information on application

Your Taxes and Savings

Jennie Hawthorne and Sally West

Explains how the tax system effects people over retirement age, including how to avoid paying more tax than is necessary. The information about savings covers the wide range of investment opportunities now available.

Further information on application

Managing Other People's Money

Penny Letts

The management of money and property is usually a personal and private matter. However, there may come a time when someone else has to take over on either a temporary or permanent basis. This book looks at the circumstances in which such a need could arise and provides a step-by-step guide to the arrangements which have to be made.

£5.95   0–86242–090–3

General

Living, Loving and Ageing: Sexual and personal relationships in later life

Wendy Greengross & Sally Greengross

Sexuality is often regarded as the preserve of the younger generation. At last, here is a book for older people and those who work with them, which tackles the issues in a straightforward fashion, avoiding preconceptions and bias.

£4.95   0–86242–070–9

Professional

Taking Good Care
Jenyth Worsley
Examines all aspects of the caring process, whether the carer is an assistant in a residential home or looking after an elderly friend or relative at home.
£6.95   0–86242–072–5

Cooking for Elderly People
Alan Stewart
Designed for use by anyone catering for groups of older people. This excellent manual contains over 120 thoroughly tested recipes.
£17.50   0–86242–046–0

A Warden's Guide to Healthcare in Sheltered Housing
Dr Anne Roberts
An invaluable guide for all wardens and care home proprietors on the health needs of older people and the best means of promoting better health for their residents.
£6.50   0–86242–052–0

To order books, send a cheque or money order to the address below: postage and packing is free. Credit card orders may be made on 081–679 8000

ACE Books
Age Concern England
PO Box 9
London SW16 4EX

INFORMATION FACTSHEETS, BRIEFINGS AND REFERENCE SHEETS

Age Concern England produces factsheets on a variety of subjects useful to Home managers as well as private individuals.

Dental Care in Retirement   Factsheet 5. This includes advice on the new dental contract and the community dental service.

Income Support for Residential and Nursing Homes   Factsheet 11. Describes financial help for an older person in need of residential, respite and convalescent care.

Probate – Dealing With Someone Else's Estate   Factsheet 14. Covers grants of representation, settling an estate, intestacy and so on.

Help With Incontinence   Factsheet 23. Includes information on buying and borrowing equipment, advice services and booklets.

Leisure Education   Factsheet 30. Advice on local and national resources, including addresses of organisations offering courses of interest to older people.

Arranging a Funeral   Factsheet 27. Includes information on arranging a funeral without a funeral director, financial help from the Social Fund, planning funerals in advance.

Ethnic Elders   A set of references on a number of topics.

Working with Older People: Activities   Selected references and organisations.

Abuse of the Elderly at Home   Selected references and organisations.

Briefing: Some financial issues for older people related to the community care reforms   An Age Concern discussion paper.

Basic Principles for working with Older People who Need Care   Single copies of this are available free; bulk copies: £5.00 per 100 from Distribution Services, Age Concern England at the address below.

To order factsheets, briefings and reference sheets

Single copies are free on receipt of a 9" by 6" sae. If you require a selection of factsheets or multiple copies charges will be given on request.

A complete set of factsheets is available in a ring binder at the current cost of £30, which includes the first year's subscription. The current cost for an annual subscription for subsequent years is £12. There are different rates of subscription for people living abroad.

Factsheets are revised and updates throughout the year and membership of the subscription service will ensure that your information is always correct.

For further information, or to order factsheets, briefings or reference sheets, write to:

Information and Policy Department
Age Concern England
1268 London Road
FREEPOST
London SW16 4BR

We hope you found this book useful. If so,
perhaps you would like to receive further
information about Age Concern or help us do
more for elderly people.

Dear Age Concern
Please send me the details I've ticked below:

other publications

☐

Age Concern special offers

☐

volunteer with a local group

☐

regular giving

☐

covenant

☐

legacy

☐

Meantime, here is a gift of

£ _____ PO/CHEQUE or VISA/ACCESS No _____

NAME (BLOCK CAPITALS) _____

SIGNATURE _____

ADDRESS _____

_____

POSTCODE _____

Please pull out this page and send it to: **Age Concern** (DEPT GCM1)
FREEPOST
1268 London Road
no stamp needed **London SW16 4EJ**

Index

training:
	for management 159-60
	for staff 11, 93, 119, 155-9
training packs and initiatives 162-3
'trial period' 33, 46, 47
trustees, appointment of 148

ulcers:
	leg 71-2, 85, 173
	stomach 74
unsteadiness 64

Validation Therapy 80, 81
Value Added Tax (VAT) 90
varicose veins 70
visiting services 133
visitors, treatment of 131-2, 148
volunteer visitors 132

Wagner Report 38, 153, 169
walking aids 64, 66
washing 122-3
waste disposal 123-4
wheelchairs 64-5, 94
White Paper *see Caring for People*
wills 52
wounds 71